Carla Valenology
Technician nical
Curator of Barts Pathology, ot the world's
most famous pathology museums, in 2011. Carla runs a blog about all
things death-related called The Chick and the Dead, and runs a dating
site for death professionals called Dead Meet. She lives in London with
her husband.

www.thechickandthedead.com
@ChickAndTheDead

Praise for *Past Mortems*

'Valentine's energy is channelled into her role as technical curator at
Barts Pathology Museum in London. Among the pickling jars you'll
find her readying 5,000 anatomical specimens for the public's gaze.
Children are welcome. By bringing the skeletons out of the attic,
Valentine has revived a once-neglected collection and enabled it to
meet the present'   Kate Womersley, *The Spectator*

'Written with cheery humour and pathos, but every so often it draws us
up with shock. A bit like death, really'   Jad Adams, *Literary Review*

'A fascinating portrait ... one seriously intriguing read'   *Glamour*

'*Past Mortems* is an engaging, brave and informative insight into
the life of those who work with death. Carla Valentine gives us a
fascinating glimpse into a life after death that is often shielded from us.
It is a reassuring guide to what may happen to us and our loved ones
after our final breath. The care, dedication and consideration given to
our loved ones mortal remains by those who work in the post mortem
world shines through on every page'   Dr Kathryn Harkup

'Today, as technical curator of the pathology museum at St
Bartholomew's Hospital, London, Valentine is one of the loudest,
liveliest and brashest advocates for confronting our modern day
taboo of death. With her striking red hair and red lipstick, her
penchant for vintage fashion and gothic tattoos, she is the antithesis
of the archetypal sombre-suited, solemn-faced male attendants of the
undertakers' world'   Wendy Moore, *Guardian*

CARLA VALENTINE

Past Mortems

LIFE & DEATH BEHIND MORTUARY DOORS

WITHDRAWN

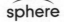

SPHERE

First published in Great Britain in 2017 by Sphere
This paperback edition published in 2018 by Sphere

A CIP catalogue record for this book
is available from the British Library.

ISBN 978-0-7515-6534-8

Typeset in Minion by M Rules
Printed and bound in Great Britain by
Clays Ltd, St Ives plc

Papers used by Sphere are from well-managed forests
and other responsible sources.

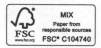

MIX
Paper from
responsible sources
FSC® C104740

Sphere
An imprint of
Little, Brown Book Group
Carmelite House
50 Victoria Embankment
London EC4Y 0DZ

An Hachette UK Company
www.hachette.co.uk

www.littlebrown.co.uk

FOR JONNY, TIL DEATH US DO PART

Contents

Author's Note

When I was a child growing up in a small city, seeing animals flattened at the roadside was a common occurrence. Frequently they would be wild creatures such as birds, squirrels, rats and even the odd hedgehog. But sometimes they were larger animals and clearly beloved pets: cats, for example, or rabbits which had managed to escape the confines of their hutch and garden only to be hit by cars; sad metaphors for the idiom 'out of the frying pan, into the fire'.

I don't seem to witness this phenomenon any more. Just like custard and scraped knees, the majority of roadkill in my life seems to have been experienced before I reached double figures. But, despite its regularity, there's still one case I remember in particular.

It was a cat, at the point of the road where the tarmac meets the kerb, and unlike most roadkill – squashed, two-dimensional testaments to the fleeting nature of life – this one was still fairly intact and, I hoped, perhaps alive. On closer inspection the injury was mainly confined to the cat's head. One eye was closed and slightly encrusted with dried blood. The other, like an early *Looney Tunes* animation, was wide open and popping out of the socket as though it had seen something alarming. It probably had: the car speeding towards it.

If it was still alive I might have been able to help it, so I picked up a nearby stick and prodded its chest. To my surprise, a small bubble of blood began to balloon from one nostril until it reached the size of a marble and popped. I experienced a moment of hope, but then I realised the cat was not alive. I knew, even at that age, it was simply residual air leaving the lungs via blood-bubble. There was nothing I could do for it now.

Or was there?

I had no reference point for the procedures surrounding death except for what I had seen on TV or read in books, but I surmised that if I was useless to this uncollared cat in life perhaps I could help it in death? Within twenty minutes I'd either knocked on the doors of my local friends or called them on their landlines (this was a long time before children had mobile phones of their own) and assembled about eight of us for a funeral procession. We moved the cat to my garden where we proceeded to dig a grave, bury the animal, say a few words and even take it in turns to sprinkle handfuls of earth on to its lifeless body – just like I'd seen people do on TV. I felt better knowing we had tended to the poor creature; knowing he or she was somewhere safe, somewhere I later marked with a little wooden cross made out of two ice lolly sticks.

Through my bedroom window, that cat continued to serve as a reminder that life can be difficult to navigate and in death it helps to know exactly what to do, whether professionally or ritually. It's how I came to feel I had a purpose.

This book contains names and identities that have been

changed to protect the privacy of the staff and patients I encountered over the years, with many tales and conversations made up of remnants from various incidents. However, it is the truth. It is also a chance to thank those who helped me bury that cat and find my path in life, as well as those I subsequently met who helped steer me along my path in death.

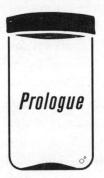

The First Cut

Anorexic. Dentist.

They were two words I'd never seen written together before but there they were, in black smudged ink, on the 97A:

'Anorexic dentist'.

I took a sip of my coffee while perusing the rest of the paperwork. I enjoyed this part of the morning: the calm before the storm. The mortuary's senior technician, Jason, was happily hunched over the latest edition of the *News of the World* with a cup of tea. As a veteran technician, he had seen it all, and he appeared less interested in the information we received on the day's cases than in the plot of *EastEnders* or the latest football scores.

The 97A is the form faxed to the mortuary from the local Coroner's Office which simultaneously requests and gives permission for the post-mortem of the deceased. Although these forms have different names in different areas, one thing remains the same all through the UK (except Scotland), and that is the Coroner gives permission for an autopsy to take place (in Scotland it's the Procurator Fiscal).

The role of the UK Coroner is constantly misunderstood because of the abundance of TV shows and crime books which continually hit our shores from the US. In America, although it varies from state to state, a coroner is another term for what we'd call a pathologist: a doctor who carries out autopsies. They're often elected in the US and in smaller states may even be the neighbourhood mortician or GP. In the UK, they are independent judicial officers appointed by the local government as a sort of overseer of all deaths in the area, and they must be qualified barristers or solicitors. Some also have a medical degree.

The term coroner comes from 'crowner', a position that has existed here formally since the year 1194. The Crowner had two roles: to oversee deaths in the area, and to be informed of any treasure that may have been discovered by a lucky serf and decide if it really was going to be 'finders, keepers' or if it belonged to someone else. This means that our Coroners sometimes have the unusual responsibility of investigating long-forgotten objects or money found buried in the garden and declaring them 'Treasure Trove'; that is, valuables of unknown ownership which become the property of the Crown. (In 1996 'Treasure Trove' became the Treasure Act.) Basically, 'whatever you find buried under your patio, be it a body or a bag of gold coins, you call the Coroner'.

I always imagine them as Grim Reapers in suits with Filofaxes and mobile phones, aware of all the deaths in their jurisdiction and poised to move all the relevant par-ticipants around like pieces on a chessboard, in order to begin the death investigation: the police, the pathologists, their Coroner's Officers, mortuary staff and more. You see, UK Coroners don't carry out autopsies, they only decide when one is required using various legal criteria, then sign a form to state that fact. After that, they watch the chess game unfold. It's the pathologist who carries out the autopsy or post-mortem – the two terms are interchangeable – and we, the anatomical pathology technologists, who assist.

So what are the criteria for a post-mortem examination in the UK? Essentially, you don't need one if (a) you have seen a doctor within two weeks of your death, and (b) the doctor knows the cause of death was natural.

Hospital patients don't tend to need Coronial post-mortems because the likelihood is that they will have seen a doctor every day they've been there. The same goes for patients in hospices and similar facilities. But nearly everyone else will. Perhaps a man passed out while running on a treadmill in the gym? Perhaps a woman collapsed at a bus stop? Perhaps unidentifiable remains were found in the park by the clichéd man walking his dog? These will all be Coronial cases that will come into the mortuary from the local area. In fact, a person may be eighty years old and die in her sleep but if she hasn't seen a doctor within the last two weeks she will still need a post-mortem. 'Old Age' doesn't tend to be written as a cause of death on death certificates any more thanks, in part, to Harold Shipman, the notorious serial killer whose victims were usually pensioners. After he was brought to trial in 1999 more than 250 victims were attributed to him and this caused a cultural shift in GP practices and death certification as well as a huge rise in post-mortem requests.

Our forms, the 97As, arrived around eight thirty in the

morning with a flurry of beeping, buzzing and swooshing as the sheets were spewed from the mouth of the ancient fax machine and on to the floor of the small mortuary office. On the pages were some details of the deceased and the salient features of the case – whatever the assigned Coroner's Officer had been able to find out in the first few hours after the death. Sometimes there were reams and reams of difficult-to-read lines, especially if medical notes were included. There might be information on prior illnesses, previous drug use, where and how the body was found, family members, charts, height and weight, and whether or not the deceased preferred one lump or two in his tea. In other cases there might be just a few words or lines, like this one:

Anorexic dentist
45 yrs
Bedridden 2 wks
Son Of a Bitch

'Bloody hell, that's harsh!' I said to Jason, so loudly that he nearly spilled his cuppa as he lifted it towards his lips.

'What is it, hun?' he asked, his eyes flying to me and away from the pages of his newspaper. He always called me 'hun' and I didn't mind. His huge, muscular, tattooed form belied a very gentle and protective nature.

'The poor bloke's dead and they're calling him a son of a bitch!'

I stomped across the office to wave the 97A in front of his perplexed face. He halted my hysterical form-flapping to get a good look at the info, and after a beat of silence and a confused expression, he roared with laughter. His massive shoulders heaved, his face reddened, and he even wiped a tear from his eye. 'Son of a bitch ...' He repeated it a few times, the words barely audible through his laughter.

When he calmed down, I discovered the reason. Although I'd read the form that way, it actually stated:

Anorexic dentist
45 yrs
Bedridden 2 wks
S.O.B.

And S.O.B. meant 'shortness of breath' No wonder Jason was in hysterics. I was going to have to get used to acronyms if I was to make it in this game.

As there was only one 97A that day, and therefore only one post mortem or PM (another acronym – *you'll* have to get used to them too), Jason said today would be my first attempt at making the incision into the deceased myself. As a trainee APT (anatomical pathology technologist – another one!) this is the first stage in learning the art of evisceration – the medical term for removing the organs, which sounds marginally better than 'disembowelling'.

Though I was only a trainee, I had the hang of the basics by now – the paperwork, signing in new bodies, carrying out viewings, small procedures like removing stubborn jewellery or false teeth – but it was time to start some proper training. It was time to do my first full incision and open the deceased. I really wanted to, I was so incredibly excited, but at the same time I was terrified. I'd wanted to do this job for so long, but now that I was about to take the plunge I suddenly had no confidence in myself. What if I messed up? What if I was no good at it and my whole life was a lie? I couldn't even cut paper straight without drawing a line with a ruler first; how was I going to cut *skin* straight? And I absolutely, positively couldn't sew any sort of fabric, so how was I going to sew a person together? Considering I'd never really been interested in paper crafts or textiles at school, the idea of trying out these little-used skills on a human being was beginning to freak me out.

To keep myself calm, I decided to focus on the things I did know, the tasks I carried out every single morning after arriving at work around seven thirty, and I realised it was only a few weeks ago I hadn't known how to do them either. I was learning quickly and I needed to stop stressing out. Everyone has to start somewhere.

So I took charge. Jason followed to observe as I headed into the small, bright post-mortem room and pulled on some latex gloves, taking a deep breath as I did so. I located the body bag of the anorexic dentist in the fridge by his name written on the door (the fridge being otherwise known as a temperature-controlled storage facility but, eager to avoid yet another acronym, we just called it a fridge). I gently slid his tray out and on to the hydraulic trolley, then I hesitated, thinking I'd made a mistake. The tray was so light it didn't seem like there was anyone actually in the bag. However, on closer inspection I could discern the curve of the top of a head pressing against the white plastic and a sharper point, much lower down, which looked like it could be a bent knee. Satisfied he was definitely in there, I took another deep breath and turned the trolley a full 180 degrees to position the tray over the stainless-steel holder jutting from the post-mortem room walls. Via this set-up the tray the deceased rests on in the fridge also becomes the dissection bed, cradled in the strong steel arms of the holder.

Sometimes the difficult manoeuvre would be done without a hitch; just the gentle glide of the turning trolley then the muted squeak of the trolley's mechanism as it lowered the tray down on to its holster.

This wasn't one of those times.

A combination of my earlier anxiety and Jason watching me intently meant I was just too nervous. There was a crash of metal on metal as I missed the turn by a couple of inches and slammed into the jutting arm with the trolley. It was nothing that would damage the deceased or even the equipment, only my ego, which was feeling more and more like it would need its own post-mortem by the end of the day: cause of death – extensive bruising.

'Don't worry about it, hun, we all do that sometimes,' Jason reassured me. 'It's a really small PM room.' I had no idea how he could be so infinitely patient with me especially since sometimes, as a newbie, I felt like all Three Stooges rolled into one.

With no real damage done, I eventually got the tray with the body bag in position on the hoist and slowly unzipped it. Jason let me carry out the entire process as though he wasn't there, which on this occasion was absolutely fine. Normally it would take two APTs to remove the patient from the bag in a well-rehearsed and carefully choreographed manoeuvre that looks like it's anything but. It involves tipping the deceased to the side, using legs and arms like levers and fulcrums, so that the plastic can be slid beneath the body on one side; the whole thing is then repeated on the other side, and the bag can be gently pulled out and folded away. But this man was so thin I could move him on my own, with one arm, while I worked the bag out with the other, as easy as holding a baby's legs aloft while sliding a nappy out from under its bottom. I concentrated on carefully removing the man while taking deep breaths to steady my nerves.

And then I got a good look at him.

I'd never seen anything like it: he resembled a knotted white twig with a few extraneous branches and hairy bark. From the front I could see the shape of his pelvic bones clearly through his meagre flesh, and when I gently rolled him away from me to view his back, every single groove of his tailbone – or sacrum and coccyx – was visible too. Where his bones had been forcing their way through his paper-thin skin during those last bedridden weeks, angry pressure sores had formed. They were deep red and wet in appearance with yellow-green infected parts, oozing pus. At the sight of them, imaginary pain involuntarily shot through me. It was so unexpected it took my breath away for a second and left me feeling winded.

His hair was long and very dark, almost black, matted to his head and upper back in some places, yet wild in others. His nails were overgrown and yellowed and, taken with the hair and the emaciation, it seemed there was more than just anorexia going on here; I was very much reminded of Howard Hughes and other recluses with psychological problems, and wondered if the same fate had befallen the dentist. But I couldn't just keep standing there musing because Jason reminded me I had a job to do by handing me a clipboard with a paper form on it. I used the form to make notes about the man's appearance; his sunken cheekbones, matted hair, bedsores and more. I noted down as much as I could, every mole, every wrinkle, every 'is that a birthmark or a bit of dirt?', and I realised it was for two reasons. On the one hand, it was my first external exam alone so I didn't want to miss anything and look incompetent to the pathologist who'd be arriving shortly. On the other, the longer I took over the examination the longer it would be until I had to make that terrifying first cut.

Jason saw right through me and, after I'd circled the body a third time like a hungry vulture, he was having none of it. 'You don't have to mark down every wrinkle on his ball-sack, hun,' he said, handing me a PM40, the mortician's main blade.

It was time.

I bent down over my patient and tried to concentrate on his neck and clavicle, the natural curve where I would begin the incision. But all I could see was the harsh light from the overhead lamp reflecting off my blade like a strobe as my hand shook.

Just then, that overhead light reminded me of something and I zoned out again. (See what I mean? Poor, patient Jason.) When we were children, my best friend Jayne and I would put make-up on each other, as many young girls do. At that moment, I had a sudden memory of lying back all those years ago with my eyes shut tight to the light above and feeling it warm my eyelids, feeling the soft stroke of the brush on my skin as Jayne applied the make-up, and thinking, 'This must be what a corpse feels like' – which is probably something most young girls *don't* do. I was specifically thinking of scenes I'd sometimes see in films or on TV where the deceased gets 'beautified' in the funeral home for the big day. In my defence, I had just seen *My Girl*, the wonderfully poignant Macaulay Culkin film from 1991. Dan Aykroyd plays a funeral director who employs the vivacious Jamie Lee Curtis to apply make-up to the dead. She made it look like so much fun, even glamorous, and it left a kind of positive impression on me, although the ending of the film certainly did not. Even now I feel traumatised if I see a mood ring or a willow tree.* With this mental image of myself as the corpse, feeling the gentle touch of the make-up brush, I suddenly imagined the anorexic dentist could feel me. Not my touch yet, but certainly my hyperventilating and my hesitating. I was sure that he wouldn't want a blonde, uncertain neophyte waving a knife above him like a sushi chef so I firmly told myself, 'Carla – get on with it.'

And I did.

I'd seen technicians make this incision many times before and I executed it almost perfectly. Starting on the right side behind the ear I slid the blade down the side of his neck, altering the angle slightly as it travelled over the clavicle and down in a 'V' to the breastbone, the skin parting with the ease of butter beneath the sharp steel. I repeated this from the left side, a slightly more awkward angle when using the right hand, and when I reached the point of the 'V' I took the blade in a straight line down his abdomen, just circum-navigating his belly button slightly. I stopped abruptly at the pubis leaving a fairly neat 'Y' shape, which is why we call it the 'Y-incision'. There were a couple of slight deviations in the skin, but I defy anyone to cut open a human being for the first time with a blade that could take off your own finger and

---

* If you haven't seen *My Girl* I highly recommend it, not only because it's wonderful but also because otherwise that last sentence will make no sense.

not falter just a little bit. Anyway, slightly wonky lines aren't visible after they've been stitched back together during the final reconstruction.

I was quite proud of myself. I stood there breathing a sigh of relief, admiring my handiwork for an inordinate amount of time, until Jason spoke.

'Come on, Edward Scissorhands, we've still got the rest of the PM to do.'

The next stage, at this point of my training, was to relinquish the blade and observe Jason for the rest of the process. Autopsy technicians tend to learn evisceration in stages, a bit like driving. For your first driving lesson you don't get in the car, gun the engine then start parallel parking and doing five-point turns, and it's the same with autopsies. It all happens step by step.

Once the incision has been made in the chest, and the breastbone – the sternum – has been removed, there are a few different methods for systematically removing the organs for examination. The most common is often called the Rokitansky Method, though in fact it was Maurice Letulle who created what is also known as the en masse procedure in which, as the name suggests, organs are removed in one large mass. This was to be the way I would carry out an evisceration for much of my career so I watched carefully as Jason proceeded.

First, some exploration, as he used his non-cutting hand to feel behind each lung for possible pleural adhesions – parts of the lung that may be stuck to the chest wall. They can be caused by previous trauma or diseases such as tuberculosis or pleurisy. The best-case scenario was that the lungs, pink, moist and healthy, would not be attached to the inside of the cavity by adhesions and after a brief manipulation – a scooping motion – would just fall back to their original position with a gentle, wet slap. With the condition of the lungs confirmed, he tackled the bowels next, their slick, curled lengths removed in one long string to be examined later, as they were not the most important part of the organ hierarchy when it came to establishing cause of death. The bowel removal created much-needed space in the crammed body cavity so Jason returned to the lungs, using the PM40 to detach them, again with another scooping motion and two long incisions, one on each side of the spine, to release each organ. Using a similar technique, he loosened each kidney and its surrounding fat from beneath the level of the stomach and liver, and sliced through the diaphragm, which separates the organs of the thorax and abdomen. He then used the blade to make a nifty slice across the top of the lungs which effectively severed the lower part of the windpipe and the food pipe – the trachea and oesophagus – from the upper part containing the pharynx and tongue, i.e. the throat. Then, with one hand he pulled the heart and lungs down and away from the spine, while gently easing the flesh away with the blade in his other hand if it was a bit too stubborn. He continued the motion down into the abdominal cavity. Soon, he was holding aloft a mass of dripping viscera which contained most of the organs from the body cavity: the thoracic components (heart and lungs) and the abdominal organs (stomach, spleen, pancreas, kidneys and liver). He lowered the mass into a huge stainless-steel bowl and placed it on the matching steel bench countertop with a metallic thump, ready for the examining doctor.

Jason then moved on to the bladder, which was still in situ deep in the pelvis. Because the deceased clearly hadn't eaten or drunk much it was small and empty: it looked like a deflated yellow balloon as he removed it and handed it to me to place on the dissection board. I wasn't sure what 'bladder-holding' etiquette was, so I pinched it between thumb and forefinger and held it at arm's length as I transported it to the steel bench, just like a disapproving mother with a teenage boy's dirty sock.

The next stage was for Jason to move on to the head. At this point in the evisceration the pathologist, Dr Colin Jameson, arrived in his maroon Volvo – we saw him slide the vehicle into the tiny car park through the frosted windows of the PM room; a bloody, moving smudge. We always mused about his choice of car, the Volvo, said to be the safest in the world. (In fact, the Volvo V40 is still the safest car you can buy.) Was it a deliberate choice? Had carrying out autopsies on so many victims of road traffic incidents – RTIs – made him paranoid, we wondered? I left Jason continuing his work on the head while I took off some of my PPE (gotta love those acronyms: this time 'personal protective equipment') and went to meet Dr Jameson in case he wanted a coffee before getting started. It was such a small building it took me only a minute to get out of my PM room clothes and into the office just as the bell rang.

The facility had recently undergone a renovation so, small as it was, it was fairly modern inside. Our single post-mortem room had two stations for autopsies but I would later discover that many had three, four or even six, and that didn't include perinatal (baby) autopsy benches. The fridges, as in most modern mortuaries, were double-sided which meant that they formed a dividing wall in the building. Behind their pristine white doors the heads of the deceased pointed into the PM room – the so-called 'dirty' or 'red' side – which is where I'd extracted this morning's patient; and the other side was the 'transition' or 'orange' side where the decedents were originally received from out in the community.* Although opening the door on that side would usually mean you were greeted by several sets of pale feet, they didn't have the proverbial toe-tags on them as you see in the media – we don't label our dead like we label our luggage. Plus the area was only for staff, never family or friends of the dead. There was also a staff office, a smaller doctors' office, a waiting room and a connecting viewing room which had the typical curtain to pull back in order to present the deceased to the next of kin.

Most mortuaries in the UK have a similar layout, particularly if they were erected in the same period. There was a spate of local authority mortuaries built in the 1950s and 1960s and they look totally unassuming from the outside, with their sharp angles, bricks and concrete. But they weren't the first mortuaries, not by a long shot. According to a paper by Pam Fisher entitled 'Houses for the Dead: The Provision of Mortuaries in London, 1843–1889' (which I consider a gripping read), the need for places to store the recently deceased was first noted in the mid-1800s. At that point London's population was booming and many families occupied only a single room, so when a family member passed

---

* Things weren't actually dirty on one side and not on the other, they're just relative terms we use for 'places where autopsies happen' and places where they don't. We also have 'clean' areas which never have any contact with the deceased, such as the office or break room. Those areas, in the 'traffic light system', are described as 'green'.

away, the decaying body was simply kept in that same room with everybody until the burial; there was nowhere else to put them. The deceased might remain there for a week or more, particularly if poorer families had to scrape the money together for a funeral, and anecdotally these corpses were said to be making the population sick. According to press from the time, learned men concluded that London's dead were killing the living, and eventually facilities were created which were to be 'houses for the immediate reception, and respectful and appropriate care of the dead'. The facilities were known as Waiting Mortuaries or Dead Houses.

When I opened the door of our own Dead House in answer to the bell, I was surprised to see someone else on the step in place of the pathologist, who was still standing at his Volvo, searching for something in the boot. It was a young police officer who appeared far more surprised to see me. He stared at me wide-eyed and in silence, looking a bit pale.

'Yeees?' I asked, slowly and deliberately, eyebrows raised, trying to encourage him to speak. It was nothing new to me: I'd been told before that first-time visitors to the mortuary expect to come face to face with a lazy-eyed male hunchback when the door creaks open, not a petite blonde Marilyn Munster. It probably caught him off guard for a second, although it didn't explain why he looked so pale. I suddenly became worried that perhaps I had a blob of fat or smear of blood on my face, so my hands involuntarily flew up to my cheek and started rubbing.

He eventually found his tongue. 'Is this the morgue?'

I took a deep breath. 'No, it's the mortuary,' I corrected him, unable to hide my annoyance.

Tiny pet peeve here: mortuary literally means 'house of

the dead' (hence Dead House) and has been in use for that purpose since around 1865. Morgue, on the other hand, comes from the French verb *morguer* which means 'to look at solemnly'. It hails from Paris in the late 1800s, when the deceased were on display at the Paris Morgue in Notre Dame for the locals to come and stare at or, I suppose, look at solemnly. Initially, this was so that the many decedents pulled from the River Seine or those who'd died elsewhere in the city could be identified by their family and friends, either physically or via their apparel. But this public activity became so popular that it could attract up to forty thousand visitors a day until it closed in 1907; to put that into perspective, it helps to know that the London Eye accommodated only fifteen thousand visitors a day in its heyday. (Not a lot to do in Paris back then, I take it?) While it's true that the terms 'mortuary' and 'morgue' are interchangeable, most UK technicians will never use the latter, though it's more common in the US.

After I'd put him right, the young policeman informed me he was escorting the funeral directors who were bringing in a deceased man from his home. I finally understood his pallor and assumed the scene had been pretty grim.

'There's a Volvo in the way at the moment, though,' he explained. 'Thought we'd just let you know.'

Five minutes later, when Dr Jameson had moved his car, he stood with me, Jason, the pale policeman and the funeral directors as we checked in the fridge's newest 'resident'. He'd been found in quite a common way: neighbours had begun to complain about a smell and flies had congregated in the area so the police had broken down his door. This didn't bode well as it meant he was very likely a recluse who had lain undiscovered for a long time, which in turn meant severe decomposition. The undertakers were complaining profusely, and one of them was particularly vocal.

'As if it's not bad enough that he's massive and green,' he grumbled, 'he was one of those – what do you call 'em? – hoarders.' He pronounced it 'orders'. 'Couldn't fuckin' get to him cos of all the piles-a-shite everywhere. Nearly broke me back, the son of a bitch!'

Hearing this, Jason turned to me and roared with laughter. I was hoping he'd forgotten my earlier mistake now that the pathologist was here. No such luck.

'Eh, Doc, you won't believe what Carla said this morning,' he chuckled, at exactly the same moment the man's body bag burst open and a spectacular wave of dark brown fluid hit the clean linoleum floor.

I put my head in my hands. This day was going to be longer than I thought.

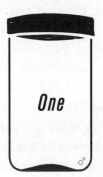

Information: 'Media Most Foul'

We live in a society in which spurious realities
are manufactured by the media. I ask in my
writing, 'What is real?'

—*Philip K. Dick*

I have never been close up to a fake corpse before. I've seen thousands of genuine cadavers in different shapes and sizes, their bouquet of smells and spectrum of colours all competing for my attention. But, in a bizarre inverse to the experience of most of the population, it's the fake corpses I'm unfamiliar with.

The prosthetic dead body now in front of me is quite pleasant despite being very realistic: she's a slender female with ivory skin and a tiny waist which I find myself envying, in the same way a young girl may envy the curves of a Barbie doll. Her long, tousled, chestnut hair is splayed around her head on the post-mortem table like a dirty halo. Her chest has been opened via the usual Y-incision, causing her loose skin to cascade over her breasts like two bloodstained pink and yellow petals, and the pearly white of her intact breastbone is just visible in the gap. She is a fake cadaver at the phase of the autopsy in which she is not quite open but merely on the cusp – just at the point where I'd relinquished my PM40 to Jason during my first case. As a result, she is still easy for me to identify as a young female and therefore identify with: the tangles of her hair immediately make me think of the struggle I have when blow-drying mine, and her fingers, curling gently up from the surface of the metal, have such a realistic human quality I'm glad they're not painted with nail polish as it would only add to the illusion. She looks so real I feel there should be an odour of blood, day-old perfume and sweat about her. There isn't, of course.

'What do you think?' the assistant director, John, asks me.

'She's wonderful,' I reply with awe. 'If only all my cases were this pleasant!'

I'm in a small, freezing-cold film studio in East London. I've been brought in because the picture being made here focuses specifically on an autopsy and the director wants to make sure everything – every instrument, every technique, every sentence – is absolutely perfect.

I have to hand it to them: as far as fake mortuaries go – and I've seen a fair few now – they've done incredibly well. There's only the odd anomaly. For example, in place of rib shears, the specific medical tool which would be used to remove that as-yet-unopened rib cage, there is a pair of heavy-duty bolt cutters from a hardware store. I suppose they do look fairly similar so they'll pass for correct. Instead of post-mortem twine, which should be more like the thick white string used to tie up parcels, there is thin green cotton – cotton which would slice through the delicate skin of a real cadaver and be useless at sewing up any incisions. Also, on a magnetic tool rack above the sink there seems to be a cake slice. I can think of no justification for that . . .

Perhaps these are things that only someone qualified to work in this environment – a pathologist or a pathology technician – would notice in a film. But, boy would they notice. 'What's a friggin' cake slice doing next to the knives and scissors?' I can already hear that audience cry, incredulous. Granted, there are some pathological conditions with confectionery-themed nicknames, such as 'maple-syrup urine disease', 'nutmeg liver' and 'icing-sugar spleen' – an observation that once led me to a pop-up anatomical cake shop called Eat Your Heart Out – but I don't think there's such a thing as 'Victoria sponge pancreas', even if it does sound delicious. Mind you, there are times when the skin of the deceased flakes off like the pastry of a croissant, and there can sometimes be a dark brown, gritty purge fluid we call 'coffee grounds' which escapes from the mouth and nose. Perhaps these, along with 'foamy discharge' and the aforementioned 'nutmeg liver', mean the dead can resemble a Starbucks menu more than a cake stand?

I do my best to explain to John that these errors will be noticeable to certain parts of the audience but he informs me it's too late now to make any changes to the props or the set because the team have already started filming scenes in the fake mortuary. I discover that in showbiz parlance this is 'the shots have already been established'. But there are still some things I can advise on: for example, the exact technique for crunching through the ribs (you really need to put your weight behind the shears and give it some welly) or the type of container that would be used to collect specimens for examination.

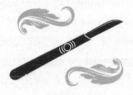

Back in the post-mortem room, after our distraction, I'm just in time to help Jason collect specimens from the anorexic dentist.

'Carla, can you swab the decubitus ulcers, please?' Dr Jameson asks.

I look at him, puzzled.

'The bedsores,' he explains.

I feel like an idiot.

Jason gently tilts the deceased on his side while I take a swab – the correct container for this type of specimen collection – from the stainless-steel cupboard and begin labelling it, hiding my flush of embarrassment behind the cupboard door. The swab's casing is a long, thin plastic tube with a rounded bottom and a blue lid. The rounded end is filled with a nutrient jelly that allows microbiological cultures to be grown and then examined in the lab. When I pull off the lid, the swab comes with it, its end already moist and prepared with the jelly from the bottom of the tube. It looks like an elongated wet cotton bud. I use this to gently swipe at some of the greenish-yellow pus in the purulent bedsores, then place the swab and its contents safely back in the tube.

Dr Jameson writes on his clipboard as he explains, 'I thought perhaps heart failure may have been his cause of death, but now I'm suspecting septicaemia.'

Septicaemia is often called blood-poisoning or sepsis and is caused by an infection entering the bloodstream. It looks as though this man's bedsores have become infected and, left untreated for so long, the microorganisms have poisoned his blood. Jason has already taken some blood samples and now they're also off to the lab for the microbiologists to help in the post-mortem process. We've done our part perfectly, for now.

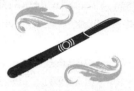

Skip forward a few years and here I am in the film studio, advising John that some of the containers they have in the fake mortuary aren't perfect but they will probably do. However, I do draw the line at one thing: this wonderful prosthetic corpse they've had made to resemble the actress Olwen, who plays the deceased main character, has something wrong with its forehead. Questioning this while bending down and looking closer, I learn that the production team assumed that brains are removed at autopsy by lopping off the top of cadavers' heads in one fell swoop – skin, skull and all. Picture, if you will, the scene from the film *Hannibal* in which Anthony Hopkins eats the brain out of the live, but drugged, Ray Liotta, and it looks a bit like a flat pink cactus in a plant pot. That's what the crew envisaged as part of the autopsy.

I stand up in disbelief and explain to John that there's a vast difference between their idea and what we actually do during the procedure. The imagery they clearly have in their heads is one of a kitsch Frankenstein's monster with his horizontal forehead slash and exaggerated stitches. Do the general public really assume that when we carry out an autopsy we access the brain via the deceased's forehead then roughly stitch it back together with thick black string? Do they think that sometimes, if the mood takes us, we throw in a couple of neck bolts too?

It makes me worry about the reputation morticians and anatomists have in general – as if members of the public never really got past the idea that we all look and act like a mad scientist's assistant named Igor, hell-bent on mutilating corpses and storing bits of them in jars for no reason other than to create a cupboard full of pathology-themed lava lamps. Films like *Re-animator* and *Young Frankenstein* give the tongue-in-cheek impression that dissection and organ retention are done for nefarious and selfish purposes such as trying to discover the secret of everlasting life or create the perfect woman, and not for the greater good.

Does it matter? Well, one would hope that when laymen read crime procedural novels or watch forensic-based TV shows they could separate reality from media fantasy and understand that sometimes clichés are perpetuated by writers or producers because they lend a certain dramatic or sexy element to an otherwise mundane scene. Obvious examples are the attractive women of *CSI* attending crime scenes with their perfectly styled hair waving in the breeze created by the fan placed at the edge of the set – and don't get me started on their low-cut tops and high-heeled shoes. Everyone knows that in real life CSIs (crime scene investigators) and SOCOs (scene of crime officers) have to wear white Tyvek suits and masks to prevent their own DNA being transferred to the crime scene, don't they? Unfortunately, not everyone does, and when there are production companies working to create drama these seemingly harmless additions and artistic licences carelessly perpetuate the macabre or simply lax reputation of mortuaries and their staff.

Around ten years ago, when I was a trainee at the Municipal Mortuary, the team was approached by a production company to be filmed for a TV series called *The Death Detective*. It was to feature a wonderful pathologist I worked with at the time called Dr Dick Shepherd.* We were happy and honoured to be filmed because the topic of autopsy was to be tackled scientifically, but only as long as the families of the autopsy cases, as well as the local Coroner, also gave consent. Surprisingly, everyone who was asked agreed and the documentary went ahead. The one thing my manager Andrew stipulated was a chance to see the final edit of the TV series before it went on air. It turned out that was a necessary and useful request. In the programme, during post-mortem room footage of one of us removing the top of the skull of the deceased to access the brain, images of our pristine mortuary floor were removed from the VT and instead a scene of blood splashing on some random tiles was spliced in. We all looked at each other in shock. Apparently, my fastidious efforts

---

* He is on TV now, in a popular programme called *Autopsy*, which examines the recent deaths of famous people. Brittany Murphy and Whitney Houston have been featured.

with the Bioguard detergent were not quite right for this production and only a blood bath would do for their visuals. However, apart from that one issue, which was corrected, the documentary did come out very well.

I'd been surprised at how many families had granted permission for filming. We'd thought it would be a battle, but next of kin were clearly curious to see what on earth goes on behind those closed mortuary doors. Some also rationalised that if their loved one's pathological findings were described to a viewer who was perhaps experiencing similar symptoms it could even encourage them to visit a doctor: televising autopsies could literally save lives.

It's exciting for anyone to be on TV, but for me, as a trainee APT, doing the job I'd always wanted to do and being able to show it my family and friends, it was as thrilling as hell. I remember inviting everyone round to my flat and making popcorn when the first episode was due to be aired. We all crowded around the screen, most people sitting on the floor and me squeezed between two more on the sofa. Everyone munched in near silence after the opening credits had rolled. There was a voiceover introduction and the first few clips, then suddenly me, tiny and blonde with a huge pair of silver rib shears, cracking my way through a man's rib cage, the tough bones making the most awful noises in the echoey post-mortem suite.

Nine astonished faces turned to me in silence in that living room, popcorn-filled hands paused halfway to open mouths.

'What?' I exclaimed as I looked from one set of wide eyes to another.

It seems my friends didn't quite understand the exact nature of my work. I suppose many of them never really wanted to think about it. That is, until they saw the brute force required and became aware that I really did have to get in there and get my hands (and arms and elbows) dirty. One of them said, 'I thought you just did paperwork or something!' and another, 'I thought you put make-up on them!' – fairly common misconceptions. With this documentary there were certainly no more unanswered questions: nothing was left to the imagination.

Correcting these mistakes matters to me because we pathology staff do our best to maintain an air of dignity during what could be considered quite an invasive and undignified procedure. The post-mortem room is as respectful and clean as most operating theatres and we want families to know that, not to watch TV and have all their greatest fears and ghoulish imaginings about autopsies and death realised.

So I'm being incredibly picky on the set of this film, refusing to let the team portray APTs as forehead-chopping miscreants. It turns out the production team would need to replace the prosthetic's entire head at a cost of hundreds of pounds if they're to show the brain removal the correct way, but I won't budge! I've developed a wonderful rapport with the special effects girls, one of whom actually used to be a SOCO before moving into SFX make-up in hospital dramas such as *Holby City*. She completely understands the dangers of misrepresentation in the media so we spend a lot of time chatting about TV shows such as *Silent Witness* and *Waking the Dead*. It's nice to have someone on set to discuss such a familiar topic with. She's of the opinion that if the current film producers were so keen on doing it right they should have asked for the guidance of someone like me long before they started creating the prosthetics and decorating the mortuary set. I have to agree with her. Getting the right information before any action is the best strategy, which is why we read through the 97A form carefully before we begin an autopsy and ensure we're fully prepared.

Exactly like the SOCO-turned-SFX girl, I too have had a career change by the time I'm on set. Although I carried out autopsies for years, eventually qualifying as a Senior in the field, I began to realise I was doing more paperwork and less hands-on pathology. That's why I'm now the technical curator of a pathology museum, and instead of opening the recently deceased and removing their pathologies for the doctors to examine, I maintain and utilise five thousand preserved examples of pathologies that have already been removed over the last two hundred and fifty years and kept for posterity in beautiful containers or 'pots'. I use these unusual objects from the human body to teach students and engage the public with the topics of medical history, the autopsy process and more. The irony is that being an APT is a very demanding job, so much so that when I did it I didn't have the time to talk about it. Now that my schedule is marginally less hectic (read that as 'bloody') I'm able to think back on and revisit all those years of training to help advise students and the public on the career via TV, theatre, writing and, of course, the current film.

A few days later I return to the set and, while the team are busy being briefed near the audio-visual equipment in what they call their 'video village', I hang back at the breakfast table to grab my coffee and brioche, avoiding any flaky pastry items of course. It's a routine to which I'm getting fairly addicted by this point. 'Chocolate chips? In the *morning*? Don't mind if I do!' I think as I reach out to the buffet. It feels very transgressive because I normally have a green smoothie for breakfast – a smoothie which also resembles some kind of post-mortem emanation, but I think that's enough food comparisons for one chapter.

Once I've stuffed the brioche in my mouth and devoured it as though my life depended on it, I decide to sneak on set and take a look around the mortuary. I enter undetected and there she is, lying on the PM table, the lovely prosthetic corpse of the star of the film. Coffee in hand, I bend over to inspect her forehead and note that the visible slash – where her head was supposed to split apart – has gone. It's good that they sorted it over the last few days, I think. I take a look again. She's so realistic, even the eyelashes! And the little hairs on the arm! I idly wonder how much she must have cost while I give her upper arm a squeeze.

She sits up.

She howls so loudly and unexpectedly that I throw my coffee so far upwards it hits the makeshift ceiling. I scream three, maybe four times in a row before we both burst out laughing at my utter idiocy and at the terrified pale faces of the crew who have run on to the set in abject horror at the sounds we made.

Of course it's not the prosthetic, it's Olwen, who is a method actress lying on the stainless-steel PM table trying to get in the right frame of mind to – well, be a good corpse, I suppose. That is, until I wandered in, bleary-eyed and curious, and decided to fondle her. I've never laughed so hard in my life. The crew and I are in tears, ribs practically splitting.

'Well, what a pathology expert I am,' I think, unable to tell a live body from a fake dead one. 'Who can't tell fantasy from reality now?'

One thing I like about the film's two main stars – both veteran Hollywood actors – is that they keep saying they're very pleased to have me there, although there is a bit of confusion about exactly who or what I am.

'It's so great to have a pathologist here!' said Emile Hirsch on my first day, shaking my hand enthusiastically.

'Thanks,' I'd mumbled shyly, 'but I'm not a pathologist, I'm a pathology technician.'

'What's the difference?' he'd asked, confused, at the same time as John said, 'But I thought you were a pathology *technologist.*'

'The pathologist is a qualified medical doctor who uses his knowledge to diagnose cause of death by dissecting the organs and examining the body,' I explained to them both. 'I offer technical support for the procedure, but I'm qualified in a different way. I carry out all the physical aspects, like removing organs and specimens, but I also help the pathologist with the diagnosis and run the mortuary.' Then I turned to John specifically. 'There are so many different words for our job but the professionally used acronym is APT. The "technician" part was changed to "technologist" a while back but it never sat well with me because the dictionary definition of "technician" makes much more sense in this context than "technologist" does.'

'Ah, I see,' they both said, with a smile.

I wasn't sure they did see. 'Look, if "technician" was good enough for R. A. Burnett, MBChB, FRCP, FRIPH, FRCPath, who literally wrote the book on the subject, then it's good enough for me!'

I laughed, realising that if a person has never seen *The Red Book*, which is basically the APT's training bible, then that joke isn't funny.

'Just call me a mortician,' I relented, embarrassed, 'for ease.'

I use the word mortician all the time though I know some other APTs don't really like it.* I use it for several reasons. Firstly, nobody knows what an APT is. If I'm asked what I do and I say I'm an APT it just stops the conversation dead (pun not intended) for all the wrong reasons, or alternatively far too many questions follow: questions about what it stands for, how you spell it, am I a doctor etc. Secondly, the official phrase 'anatomical pathology technologist' is incredibly clunky – my tongue wraps around it like a thrashing eel. I think 'mortuary technician' is neater and self-explanatory, but I like to imagine the words 'mortuary' and 'technician' as two separate, cumbersome handfuls of snow which I can squeeze into one compact snowball of a word: 'mort-ician'. Everyone knows what 'mortician' means. Then, like a snowball, it can be metaphorically thrown into the face of the enquiring person in a cold, descriptive burst which surprises them and makes them shake their head in disbelief.

But finally, I'm not only an APT: my career with the dead has spanned embalming, medical dissection and prosection, excavation and examination of bones as well as

---

* I'm not sure why there's such haughtiness about it. I meet people all the time who say 'I'm a nurse' not an 'SRN' (state registered nurse) or 'I'm a doctor' not an 'SpR' (specialist registrar). It's just more conversational and casual to use terms people are familiar with. There's nothing wrong with that.

conserving historical human remains. As an individual I *am* a mortician.

'Really? A *mortician*? You don't look like one!' is the usual response. And I quite like that; I like being something totally different from what my exterior implies. But more than that, I've worked with the dead all my adult life and it is important to me to get that passion across. It's become part of my identity. As the poet-undertaker Thomas Lynch described it, I am one of the 'people whose being had begun to meld with their doing'. Me the person and Me the caretaker of the dead are two entities that have become indivisible.

I had already met the older of the two actors, Brian Cox, as he had previously been to the Pathology Museum where I work to record part of a documentary he was presenting. That particular segment was all about the dangers of alcohol on the liver and I'd had to bring a variety of livers to the table and present them for the crew's approval. It was a bit like being a London market trader, setting down my wares and trying to convince them of their quality so I didn't have to keep hauling livers all over the place from three different floors:

'Nah, this is a lahvly liver, mate, exactly wotcha lookin' for.'

'Nah, sir, ya don't want that one up there – I'll do y'a deal on this one!'

He and Emile, who is playing the part of Brian's son, both seem jovial enough at first, and the crew keep reminding me I'm a necessary part of the team: 'Brian and Emile are so pleased you're here to help them out.' That is until week four of the shoot when they are getting tired and acting like the typical divas you imagine from the tabloids. Emile is growing more and more irascible and Brian seems to have lost interest and comes back on set after the lunchtime break looking anything but enthusiastic. The crew asks me to work some more days but, apart from the fact I really don't want to be *anywhere* for twelve hours a day, let alone a freezing-cold warehouse studio, I just can't spare the time away from my day job. On my final day I ask the art director if the actors' behaviour is typical of a film because I don't really have a clue and she says, 'No, it's just been a very "trying" project.'

I witness this first hand when, on my last day, I offer some advice to Emile and he shouts at me, 'Nobody will know and *nobody cares.*'

'Oh, well, I'm glad I've been spending twelve hours a day here to advise you on correct procedure, then,' I think as I quietly walk away.

I wonder again whether this is reflective of the attitude of others: that somehow what we do in mortuaries is considered so weird or unimportant that nobody cares anyway and no one wants to know. There's a definite divide between people who enjoy this type of work or want to know all about it, and people who think it's totally bizarre. I can't count the number of times someone in the crew whispered to me, 'A film set – it's exciting, isn't it?' and I had to whisper back, 'No, it's a bit boring. To me this would be more exciting if it were a *real* mortuary and a *real* autopsy.' I chose to work with the dead because I find it interesting and incredibly rewarding. Hanging around on productions, for me at least, is not really how I'd prefer to spend every day.

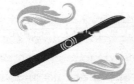

Conversely, in the post-mortem room, the action never stops. Even though the pathologist has left there is still work to be done. Jason has taken on the cleaning so that I can focus on reconstructing the anorexic dentist. I sew all his incisions together, I wash him, I comb his unkempt hair, I place dressings on his bedsores and I even trim his overgrown fingernails. He actually looks better now than when he first came in. He's perfectly viewable for any family or friends ... but no one has come forward to ask to view him. It's not a wasted effort, though; I did this for him, not necessarily for anyone else. That's why it's rewarding – he looks at peace now. I gently graze his forehead with my hand to make sure his eyes are properly closed, then zip up the body bag and place him back in his section of the fridge.

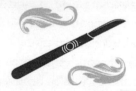

Many people do think working with the dead is interesting and want to know more so I give a lot of interviews. The problem with giving interviews is that even with the best intentions, writers can alter what you've said for dramatic effect, or not do their research correctly. It's not because they're being malicious – death inhabits a very confusing and sensitive world.

Take the dead body, for example. I can euphemistically call the deceased someone's 'loved one' or a 'decedent'. In certain contexts, for example when we study taphonomy (the science of decaying organisms) or discuss organ and body donation and dissection, we refer to the dead as 'cadavers'. The word 'patient' just wouldn't make sense. Yet when I worked in a hospital mortuary they were all called 'patients' because they came to us from the hospital and the autopsy is the last part of their medical journey, so they're still technically under patient care. However, those who work in Coronial mortuaries, like I did at first, don't use the term 'patient' and are more likely to say 'case'. They all mean the same thing but they have their own individual nuances which don't quite make sense in all contexts, and a journalist, for example, may not understand that. That is why I try my best to give thorough interviews when anyone is kind enough to ask me to, but it can't be helped if *my* use of the word 'patient' gets changed to 'corpse' in the final edit because of the perceived confusion it may cause for the reader.

And everyone is especially interested in dead people or body parts or 'remains' or 'cadavers' at Halloween; I become particularly popular around that time of year. I always thought my fifteen minutes of fame were done and dusted with *The Death Detective* and never really expected any more front-of-camera brushes with showbiz until I was asked to go on Alan Titchmarsh's show and bring some specimens from the Pathology Museum. The segment was to be on bizarre medical cures through the ages, one of my favourite topics, since many of the specimens in the pathology collection illustrate them. For example, there are syphilitic bones, twisted and pocked, from people who'd not only suffered with the infection but also from the damaging effects of the toxic mercury used as a 'cure'. There is also a pot containing a long, thin tapeworm, an example of something women used to deliberately swallow as a diet aid; if you have a tapeworm living in your small intestine then it'll consume the calories and you won't . . . or so the theory goes.

I was collected from work in a taxi, carrying a plastic crate containing delicately wrapped bones, tapeworms and more. I had absolutely no idea what to expect and I was a bit self-conscious when I arrived at the studio, considering the bizarre nature of my cargo. But when I was helpfully shown to the Green Room, given a coffee and introduced to the other guests I started to relax. I needn't have thought the box of body parts was the weirdest thing happening that day because in the Green Room were Rula Lenska, some of the Muppets, the Hairy Bikers and a baby that could do the dance to Beyoncé's 'Single Ladies (Put a Ring On It)'. When my time came to get on stage and meet Alan and talk through the specimens live on camera in front of a studio audience, I just got on with it without any nervousness because I think I assumed I was dreaming.

The tactic must have worked because they invited me back on to the show for a Halloween special, this time to discuss a topic of my choosing. I talked about the medical origins of some popular monsters and brought in preserved examples of those conditions. One was leprosy as a real-life zombie analogy. Lepers used to be known as the zombies of the Middle East, declared un-dead by the Catholic Church. They were alive and yet they were not considered to be, so they had no rights. Another was porphyria, a type of anaemia, which may have given rise to the vampire myth as it leaves sufferers unable to go out in sunlight and causes their teeth to be stained red. They even asked me to take part in a quiz at the end of the show which consisted of Halloween-themed questions and tasks, and of course I won – I *love* Halloween! The prize was a golden pumpkin – a real mini pumpkin sprayed with gold paint. It was my pride and joy for about six months until one day I realised it had deflated into a bronze fungus and I knew it was time to lay it to rest. It went the way we all eventually will and decomposed into the earth. Unless, of course, we're artificially preserved in pots like those under my charge now.

The specimens were a hit on TV. Human remains have power which fakes and fabrications do not.* In the UK it is difficult for most people to have contact with real human remains for various reasons, one being that we don't tend to lay out our own dead like we used to and instead have profes-sionals do it for us. Another is that museums, such as the one I work in, containing the remains of deceased individuals, require special licences in order for the general public to be able to see them. But I feel that there are things only human remains can teach us: they have an intensity and an agency that facsimiles don't.

I remember being in history class aged about fourteen, learning about the Nazis. It seemed that half the class were more interested in spraying Impulse deodorant on them-selves and reading *Just Seventeen* so our teacher became furious with us. 'These people made lampshades out of human skin!' he shouted. 'How can you just witter on as though nothing horrifying happened?' But we couldn't relate – we were teenagers, more interested in whether or not our boobs were growing and we could upgrade from crop tops to bras than some random thing that happened in some

---

* OK, I was caught out that *one* time when I confused a prosthetic for a live human being but that's not quite what I mean.

random place years before we were born. It wasn't until I
saw a Holocaust exhibition – the piles and piles of human
hair that had been shaved off the Nazis' victims' heads – that
the horror actually hit me. There was a force from those
remains that told me they would not be ignored. Student
doctors feel the same when they dissect their designated
cadavers in the labs at our medical school; they appreciate
the donation and become attached to their charges. They
even have a ceremonial Service of Remembrance at the end
of the year once they finish their dissections. The new fake
SynDaver™ made from silicon rubber will not elicit the same
power and respect.

Actor Bradley Cooper felt the same. He played the
Elephant Man in a recent production at a London theatre,
and although there is a replica of Joseph Merrick's skeleton in our public museum he asked to see the real remains,
which reside in one of our galleries reserved only for medical
students and researchers. He wanted to do the part justice
so we obliged. He was praised for his representation of the
character of Joseph Merrick and was very respectful of his
remains. In fact, the day before he left to return home to the
US he came back to see Joseph, simply to say goodbye to him.
That skeleton is human, those decedents on the autopsy tables
are human, even the people in my five thousand specimen
pots are human. Important, powerful, and full of stories to
tell – stories that I am privileged to be qualified to elicit in
different ways.

This is why I love what I do now: the randomness of one
day being on TV wearing a badge that says 'Creepy Carla'
and winning a golden pumpkin, on another re-potting a

specimen of a hernia from 1750, then on yet another being on a film set manhandling a method actress. I have years of experience carrying out autopsies, but as I said, the irony is that back then I was so busy I could never pursue any extra-curricular activities such as furthering my studies or appearing on TV. Now that I don't work in mortuaries full time I'm much freer to reflect on what a totally crazy, rewarding and fulfilling job being an APT actually is. I have one foot in death's past with my current job and collection of human remains, and one foot firmly in death's present and future.

Working in a mortuary is not a dead-end job.

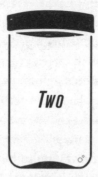

Preparation: 'Grief Encounters'

> I am prepared to meet my Maker. Whether
> my Maker is prepared for the great ordeal of
> meeting me is another matter.
>
> —*Winston Churchill*

My granddad, Frederick, gratefully took the weight off his legs and sat back into his favourite chair with a gravelly sigh which metamorphosed into a smoker's cough. We had just come in from what I called 'the garden', although it was really just a grassy patch at the front of the sheltered accommodation which he and my nan, Lily, called home. Still, it seemed like a huge garden to seven-year-old me and I can remember running lengths of it, back and forth, back and forth, as he sat with his back to the wall and his face to the sun, smoking a roll-up.

Looking back now, my granddad reminds me of Sid James, with his slicked-back grey hair and mischievous laugh which pushed his shining eyes into tight slits. But in younger years, in photos of him marrying my nan, for example, he was like Humphrey Bogart: all sharp suits and Brylcreem. During the Second World War he fought in Burma, though he never spoke about it, and he played the accordion because he was descended from Gypsies. And I don't mean the ones you see on TV now, in huge, gaudy wedding dresses wearing too much make-up. I mean the ones from the Old Country who traversed the land in brightly painted horse-drawn caravans called vardos: proper Romani Gypsies who drank unpalatable liquor by firelight, who'd curse you as soon as look at you, and who slaughtered chickens during rituals to find out which of the family's females would marry first.

My granddad's father, my great-granddad, had been a Gypsy boxer, despite having arms so short he wore garters to hold up his shirt sleeves long after they were fashionable. He had one long thumbnail, a bit like Sport from *Taxi Driver*, and he used this to mend clocks. He also pierced people's ears (no, not with his thumbnail), and he turned his one-hoop earring into a wedding ring for my great-grandmother. After they married they had five children but all of them died as was fairly common a hundred years ago. After moving to the UK in around 1903 they had another five of which my granddad, Frederick, was the eldest. This is really all I remember of my granddad's life.

More vivid in my memory is the look on his face during his death.

Just after he sank back into his comfy chair that day he began to convulse. From my vantage point at his slippered feet I looked up at my granddad but found myself staring into the face of death itself. His eyes rolled back into his tilted head and one lone droplet of blood trickled from the corner of his lips and painted a delicate crimson trail across his crêpey cheek. Then, like an exclamation point, his dentures comically shot out of his mouth and landed on the carpet with a thud. I don't remember who but somebody wrenched me away from the scene, and the implication was clear: this was something a seven-year-old child shouldn't see.

My granddad had suffered a massive stroke. He didn't technically die in that chair but he never recovered once he reached the hospital. He passed away with my mum and aunts around him. I didn't go to the funeral because I was considered too young, and I don't remember how my family behaved on that day. But I do remember one thing about his death – I had been intrigued as well as afraid.

I was quite a ballsy child and I think I inherited that from my father, a rather arrogant and headstrong man from a huge Catholic family. In me, the eldest of two children with a less rigid upbringing than he'd had, those personality traits just manifested as independence, a desire for knowledge, and a need to be frequently alone with my books or with my thoughts. I learned to read at about two years old and apparently I could tell my mum what time my favourite TV show was on by reading it in the paper. Once, when attempting to punish me, my mum sent me to my room, as all flustered parents do. After an eternity of what she considered to be 'difficult solitude' she came by to investigate and found me quietly and happily reading. 'It's OK, you can come out now,' she reassured me, to which I replied, 'I just want to finish this chapter first.' Some punishment!

My brief encounter with death may have terrified lesser children but I was of different ilk and, fascinated, I saw this enigmatic Grim Reaper as a challenge; something to research. I had an innate acceptance of the way the world worked and I understood at a young age that there could be no light without darkness.

Perhaps for that I can blame my strange pagan Gypsy blood. Perhaps it was my father's morbid Catholic influence. Perhaps blame my insatiable appetite for Agatha Christie at an age when I should have been content reading Enid Blyton. Or perhaps you could blame the Bunny Massacre.

My father would sometimes, out of the blue, gift me and my little brother random pets. Once it was two young black and white rabbits, and even though we hadn't asked for them, the last thing children do is turn pets away, especially little bunnies. So, one huge hutch and a lot of hay later, the two new rabbits were happily sheltered from the elements in their new home: the garden shed. We'd let them out of the hutch to roam around the shed every day, or watch them run free in the garden, safe in the knowledge they were protected from cats on the prowl. Or so we thought. One day, without warning, there was a cacophony of high-pitched squeaking and snarling from the garden which caused us in the dining room to freeze, forks halfway to mouths. Eventually, coming to our senses and rushing out into the bright daylight, we were assaulted by a tableau like a scene from a US sorority house movie: as though several lithe female students had just finished their sexy pillow fight, and errant feathers were now floating delicately down on to their languid, heaving bodies. Only instead of white feathers it was clumps of fur, and instead of sticking to sweaty tanned limbs they were sticking to twitching, bloody rabbit carcasses.

You see, my father had chosen a male and female rabbit and, unbeknown to us, they'd mated and she'd given birth to what seemed like a million babies. They were so tiny they'd ingeniously hidden from us in the crevices of the shed whenever we'd gone in there: between the hutch and the wall, behind the chest freezer, under the lettuce and behind the water bowl. We had no idea they even existed. It seemed that a determined cat had managed to sneak into the shed through its tiny window and had a field day, much like Mike Myers on Halloween. Before we even knew of their existence this cat had slaughtered all the little newborns, just for sport.

Well, nearly all.

Once the final clump of fur had settled and we'd raked over the carcasses like a bunch of hyenas, we did find one tiny bunny still alive and shaking. I remember being able to hold this pitiful creature in the palm of my hand because it was so small, and I recall feeling its frantic, delicate heartbeat against my skin. I felt helpless, as if I should have somehow seen this tragedy coming, and if not that, then at least be able to put it right somehow.

Death, my Old Foe, had struck again.

The more you know about something, the more you can control it. In the case of tragedy, demystifying it helps you to regain control of the emotions. I did that with death. They say 'keep your friends close and your enemies closer'. Well, I kept my enemy, Death, so close to me it eventually felt confident enough to shoot ahead, do a complete lap around, and join me once more as my friend.

*

A stroke is medically known as a cerebrovascular accident (CVA), although in some ways there's nothing 'accidental' about it. One of the main risk factors is tobacco smoking so my granddad, with his roll-up cigarettes, had contributed to his own death. Other risk factors include high blood pressure, high cholesterol and obesity – all things we can try to manage ourselves. I know this because years later, as a trainee APT, I would hold in my hands the brain of someone who had died from a CVA while Dr Jameson explained all this to me.

'A stroke occurs when blood flow to part of the brain stops, either due to a blockage or the rupture of a blood vessel. Here – you can see the rupture.' He pointed to a dark red area of blood in the pale brain slice. 'You can decrease the risk of a stroke with blood thinners like the humble aspirin and generally taking good care of yourself.'

'And can you tell if one is coming?' I'd enquired, thinking of my granddad as I carefully placed the fragile brain back down on to the dissection board.

'Yes. One side of the body may go numb or the vision in one eye may deteriorate. There might even be weakness to one side of the face and slurring of speech.'

And there it was; I felt like I'd known it or at least wanted it to be the case since the day my granddad passed away: you *could* see Death coming if you knew what to look for. You could control him.

Well, at least you could try.

The first time my mum heard I wanted to be a mortician was when I was about nine years old, in the salon chair, as the hairdresser carried out the usual ploy of chatting to me to distract me while she removed chunks of my hair, lest I start screaming.

'What do you want to be when you grow up?' she sweetly asked, to which I replied 'A mortician', just as sweetly.

I'm sure the scissors paused in mid-air at this, just for a moment, while the hairdresser glanced at my mother who returned her inquisitive stare with a shoulder shrug as if to say 'nothing to do with me'. It just wasn't that common for a small, blonde, female child to say they wanted to be a mortician in those days – the days before the media made death and forensics popular. It wasn't a career that was well known and it wasn't something that ran in my family, but for me it was a calling; I don't remember ever wanting to do anything else. I had always been fascinated by the body and how it worked, long before I associated the miracle of life with inevitable death – a lesson I had learned at my dying grandfather's feet. But after that fateful day I wanted to know what had happened to his body to snuff out his life so quickly, like a clockwork toy shuddering just before the energy is completely spent and the key stops turning.

And it didn't stop there.

I was enthralled by any dead animal I found on the street – just like that poor cat – and often roped my friends into giving them burials in the garden. This is a very common thing for young children to do when becoming aware of their own mortality so please don't worry if your little one creates a graveyard in the garden – you don't have a budding serial killer on your hands. Perhaps less commonly, though, the maggots, the blood and the bloating only piqued my curiosity rather than dampened it: I needed to know what was going on. I asked for a microscope around my tenth birthday, and on 'Bring in a Toy' day at school I did a show-and-tell about how it worked to my classmates who I imagine were less than thrilled. I'm quite surprised I had *any* friends, now that I think of it. At the same age I could often be found wandering to the local library and borrowing A-Level biology textbooks to pore through on my own. I read in one of those many books that an earthworm cut in half will become *two* earthworms. Imagine that! Like a tiny Dr Frankenstein with pigtails and knee socks, I thought this was the key to avoiding death. Worm after worm was pulled out of the undulating mounds of our garden/graveyard by my relentless little fingers, then chopped in two and observed with a magnifying glass.

My long-suffering mother was not happy with this use of her cutlery.

I still go to the hair salon, of course, and when I inevitably get asked about my job I'll happily talk about it. These days people are often very interested, and many of the other customers and stylists in the salon usually get involved in the chatter too. Everyone, it seems, has seen *CSI* or *Silent Witness*, or read books by Patricia Cornwell or Kathy Reichs and has a glamourised idea of what the job is like. Forensic science fascinates, and as long as I don't go into too much of the minutiae of my routine (nobody wants to hear about that time I walked around with faeces on my elbow all day) I can quite happily carry on a conversation for hours about work, usually being asked the same questions I've been asked a million times before. In any case, they're so much better than the usual salon queries about where I'm thinking of going on holiday. Corpses = interesting. Costa del Sol = not so much.

The exception is when I go to get my nails done (and I do this now because I was unable to when I worked in mortuaries due to the constant use of my hands for intricate work, so forgive me this one small vanity. If you'd spent eight years walking around in wellington boots and PPE looking like a fishwife, you'd do everything you could to feel glamorous now, too.) There's one man in particular at the salon I often ask to do my nails because, in a bizarre synchronicity, he has just one long thumbnail, exactly like my great-granddad, which he uses to scrape errant nail varnish from my cuticles when he makes a mistake. I never met my great-granddad but the similarity gives me comfort.

None of the nail technicians in my local salon speak much English so I can't really do anything except watch them. And I like to watch them because, as they go about their intricate work, they remind me of *me*, and of many APTs like me, as we prepared for an autopsy. They carry out their task diligently, with all their tools and all their liquids and powders ready to go – a place for everything and everything in its place. They are prepared even to the point of tearing off single pieces of absorbent paper towel so they don't need to scrabble about for it later and mess up the whole roll.

That was how I began every single day as an APT, coming into work at least half an hour before I was meant to, no matter where I was employed, and always long before the pathologist arrived. Generally, as an APT my day would start at eight but I'd arrive at seven thirty to put the coffee maker on before colleagues appeared. Because the pathologists aren't around for the whole autopsy they'd usually pop their head in to identify the deceased first and sign some paperwork before going to their office and allowing us to carry on with the preparation.

This initial identification is obviously extremely important – a decedent will be checked and checked and checked again via ankle ID and wrist ID. Carrying out a post-mortem on the wrong person would be unthinkable. Once identified, the doctor would then leave, aiming to be back down in about an hour's time, and this would be my time to shine: I'd begin the autopsy, a term which comes from the Greek 'to see oneself' or 'examination of the self'.

For me, everything had to be laid out meticulously, ready for the procedure, or I felt like I wasn't doing my job properly. I liked being the type of APT who would be holding a particular utensil or object aloft ready for the doctor before they even asked for it, like a nurse in an operating theatre. That way I felt in control of what I was doing, and that's all the better for the patient. In addition to this, post-mortems are messy and you will get covered in blood and other fluids so the last thing you want to do, when the procedure is in full swing, is open cupboard doors and drawers and start searching for things like swabs or spare scalpel blades. Much better to do what the nail technicians do and pre-empt every possible action.

First I'd ensure there was plenty of what we call 'blue roll' to hand, an absorbent paper towel we used to mop up spills and clean out cavities. I'd lay out all my tools, with fresh blades on the scalpels, and the PM40 – which is like a very large scalpel with a blade so big it needs to be screwed on – but once attached I'd leave the new blades shrouded in their foil or paper wrappers, having once been told that even the gentle action of oxygen molecules blowing against the thin blades' surfaces can dull them. I didn't know if it was true but I wasn't taking any chances with my equipment.

Other tools laid out would include a very long knife about an inch thick with a square end, a bit like a Samurai sword, called a brain knife. A sharp, disposable blade like this is necessary to slice the delicate brain into sections. There were the rib shears I've mentioned, used for cutting through the ribs at the costal cartilage, which is much softer than the bone. The older a person gets, the more calcified their cartilage becomes, and it's tougher to cut through without creating ragged edges and bone splinters which can actually penetrate your gloves and even your flesh. This is what caused such an awful noise when my friends watched me on TV. There was a ladle or two and something called a skull key which is a T-shaped piece of metal used to aid removal of the top of the skull later on. There was an array of scissors including bowel scissors, a variety of forceps (some with teeth and some not – a bit like my patients) and the cute-sounding 'bone nibblers' used for delicately removing pieces of bone. I'd also thread large, curved C- and S-shaped needles with thick white twine ready for sewing the skin together, and tape them to the side of the cupboard so they'd be ready to pull off and use. There's nothing worse than fiddling with pristine rolls of twine when you have several pairs of gloves on, slippery with blood. But I tried not to automatically do what I might if I was sewing fabric with cotton: that is, moisten the end of the string with my mouth to sharpen it to a point! Soon the tool trolley would have a DIY vibe about it too, because I'd add a chisel or two with a huge mallet, an electric bone saw as well as a manual one in case the power cut out, and several large buckets and bowls.

Although every case was slightly different, there were common procedures. I'd be able to guess what specimens would be taken from someone suspected of an intravenous drug overdose, and they'd be different from those taken from someone who died in a nursing home and had a bedsore, for example. In the former, it would be necessary to send samples of body tissue to toxicology to establish exactly what levels of which substances were present in the tissues, and whether or not they led to the cause of death. In the latter, just like in the case of the anorexic dentist, a microbiology swab would be taken as a record of the sores and what organism they were specifically infected with. In his case, it took a couple of weeks for the pathologist to receive results from the lab, and that is fairly standard – unlike on TV, when results appear within the hour. The doctor was right: the cause of death had been septicaemia leading to septic shock due to microbes entering the blood from the decubitus ulcers.

Pathologists, too, are all different, and part of the skill of being an APT is getting to know each one well enough to pre-empt the equipment they'll require. Some would be more fastidious than others, requiring many more specimens to support the conclusion they'd eventually reach. And more specimens meant more containers and labels, which would need to be pre-printed, ready to go on pot after pot of urine, blood, vitreous humor from the eye, bile, pus, tiny pieces of organs or bone and more. These small sections, taken for histology – the microscopic study of cells – were usually about a centimetre by a half and fitted neatly into plastic cases called histology cassettes. If I had a feeling the pathologist needed to take 'histo' then I'd have these cassettes out ready too, also printed with a unique case number, already with their lids open and standing to attention along the edge of the dissection board like little soldiers. Contrary to popular belief, it's not very common for a pathologist to remove and keep whole organs. Modern techniques with microscopes mean that the smallest pieces of tissue are all that are required. The exception may be if there was extensive and unique damage to tissue and in that case the doctor would receive consent to keep the specimens for whichever length of time and whatever purpose was necessary.

With all this preparation, everything was out and ready to go in order for the post-mortem to run as smoothly as it possibly could.

The mantra one of my colleagues taught me was 'the Five Ps' – Prior Preparation Prevents Poor Performance. It applies to everything in life, from cooking your beau a romantic meal to disembowelling humans. It also applies to embarking upon your chosen career. Most people don't accidentally end up in their ideal vocations, and I couldn't just fall into a job like anatomical pathology. I had to work at it and start preparing from an early age.

After the fairly restrictive years at my religious school, culminating in GCSEs, I went to college. I opted to study some Biology and Psychology but I also worked part-time as I wanted the freedom, money and time to mature a little. After working in my gap year, I did a Foundation Degree in Biological and Chemical Sciences, which was the equivalent of doing A-Levels in Biology, Chemistry, Physics and Maths in one year. This led me directly into a degree in Forensic and Biomolecular Sciences during which I'd not only learn more about the human body in detail but also the techniques used by forensic scientists. Modules I studied included toxicology, microbiology, cellular biology and forensic anthropology – the examination of skeletal and decomposed remains.

I thoroughly enjoyed being at university and working towards a goal but, having also had real work experience, I felt I wanted something more than simply sit-down lectures. I knew that reading books on forensics and autopsies was one thing and seeing images in class from an experienced pathologist or anthropologist was another, but I needed to know exactly how I would react in the presence of the most difficult cadavers; I needed the whole multi-sensory experience. If I could handle the worst, then I could handle anything. Looking at pictures of decomposing corpses is very different to smelling them and feeling the Rice Krispie pop of maggots beneath your feet.

Then fate struck when I met the eminent forensic pathologist Dr Colin Jameson, who was giving an evening lecture on Mass Grave Excavation in Srebrenica.* I commandeered his time to chat after the lecture – I was shy but what did I have to lose? In fact, he was very accommodating and I discovered he worked in several mortuaries, one of which was very near where I studied. He suggested I drop in one day to facilitate my university degree and that's how I ended up on the steps of the Municipal Mortuary asking if I could volunteer one afternoon a week. I thought I'd have no chance but, perhaps because it was very uncommon for people to want to work in mortuaries then or perhaps because Dr Jameson had vouched for me as a student, the new manager there, Andrew, said yes. I was allocated some steel-toe-capped wellington boots

---

* Yes, that was the sort of thing I did in my spare time: attended lectures on mass fatality protocol and capacity building in post-conflict regions rather than head out to the students' union for Red Bull and vodka.

of my very own and I entered the world of the mortuary, not really knowing what to expect. As much as I'd tried to research and prepare I was only really familiar with sensationalist 'morgues' from the media. Would there be organs in glass jars on shelves? Would there be stone slabs and weird electrical equipment, like something from a B-movie? Not at all – it was all very bright and clean.

Although the recent renovation of the mortuary meant everything was fairly modern, there was one throwback to the 'creepy mortician' stereotype of old: the current senior technician and lone staff member, an ageing Teddy boy. He was called Alfie and he was a real character, a relic from the days when everyone who worked in the death-business was male. He had stringy grey hair greased up into a Teddy-boy quiff and thick 1950s-style glasses which he wore non-ironically. He was originally from London and sounded just like Michael Caine, although the accent may have been slightly exaggerated.

The mortuary had been renovated because the local council had been restructured; it had been moved from the Public Health Department, which put it in the same category as Pest Control and Refuse Services (i.e. rats and bin bags), to the much more apt Cemeteries and Crematoria Services, run by the new head, Arnold. On seeing the mortuary and its staff, a decision was made by Arnold and his team that absolutely everything must go, starting immediately with Alfie's co-worker, Keith, and then, soon after I arrived, Alfie himself. When I'd been there a while and heard tales of Alfie and Keith's exploits I could understand why . . .

Because mortuaries used to come under the banner of Public Health, one worker used to use his ambiguous identification card to receive free meals at restaurants under the pretence that he was a health inspector there to grade them. Apparently, he also brought his dog to work every day and it was given free rein to wander between the office and dirty post-mortem areas at will ... and then go back to his house. He kept porn in his locker at work; another worker, Samurai swords. They ate and smoked in the post-mortem room and wore their own clothes with nothing but an apron over the top – no scrubs, no disposable gowns, nothing. The whole set-up was a health, safety and ethical nightmare.

When I was asked to pop in and chat about volunteering it was mainly discussed with Andrew, a young, serious man who slightly resembled Beaker from *Sesame Street* with his glasses, strawberry blond hair and white shirts which reminded me of lab coats. He was evidently determined to bring anatomical pathology into a new era and I can't say I blamed him. Mortuary work in particular had been undergoing an image overhaul over the course of the late nineties and early noughties, a natural progression as part of the Modernising Scientific Careers initiative. It was being championed by a younger, more progressive generation who wanted the work as pathology assistants to involve more qualifications and stringent checks – checks there's no way some of the older generation would ever have passed.

I came in every Thursday (my one day off from university), and while Andrew stayed in the office to send emails and deal with paperwork and get the mortuary's new management systems up to scratch, I went into the post-mortem room with Alfie. I watched him remove the deceased from the fridge for examination and I met the different pathologists as they arrived to carry out the autopsies, telling me their findings, which I made notes on. My little autopsy notebook was filled with exciting new fragments:

22nd Feb: myocardial infarction most common cause of death in the Western world; 29th Feb: pulmonary embolism in CALF MUSCLE! Watched Dr. J open the leg!!

I viewed all the organ dissections by the pathologists and watched as Alfie put them in a viscera bag and set them back into the body, and I observed Alfie alone as he reconstructed the decedents and placed them back into their temporary refrigerated tombs. Then I helped to clean up all the mess. I did all this in silence. I didn't really want to engage with him as, in so many ways, what he did represented the old way of carrying out mortuary work while I was more interested in the way younger APTs were attempting to change the old approach to anatomical pathology. I do remember him telling me that he had been friends with the infamous London gangsters the Krays in their heyday, and how they had thrown a dead body off a bridge over the Thames.

I just nodded politely.

Also, he told me he wanted to write and publish a book called *Death Can Be Fun*. He never did, and at the rate he was smoking when I met him, I seriously doubt he's still alive.

This continued for a year – my studying and helping out in the mortuary every week. Soon enough, Alfie was gone, replaced by the younger APT, Jason, who was working as a locum APT then. (This meant he travelled around the UK to work short stints in mortuaries which were understaffed. It could be for a week or two, or even months in the case of maternity leave, for example.) Jason was a lot of fun. He was huge because he was a bodybuilder, enthusiastic about training me in mortuary ways as well as chatting about the gym. I'd always had the romantic idea that being a mortuary technician would be like being in the FBI and assumed I'd need to be physically fit. I modelled myself on Clarice Starling from *The Silence of The Lambs* and Dana Scully from *The X-Files* and became a bit of a gym fanatic. I was in there most of the time when I wasn't in the mortuary or at university and it was a good move because I hadn't realised until I volunteered that being an APT involves a lot of time on your feet. Good strong leg and back muscles are required just for that alone, never mind the fact I had no idea at this point what sort of strength was needed to carry out an evisceration. Jason allowed me to wash the deceased myself, rather than just watch, and explained all the qualities of the different disinfectants, which I could relate to because of my microbiology studies. He also handed me bowls full of organs – the bigger the better – to help me get used to the weight, so that I constantly looked like a dinner lady at an industrial canteen heaving massive bowls of pasta around and complaining about my back.

Finally, the day came for the Municipal Mortuary to advertise for a trainee, someone like me who wanted to be a fully trained APT but had to start on the bottom rung of the ladder, with years of on-the-job training ahead and a qualification at the end of it. I had to apply for the job and go for an interview like everybody else. I met the management team from the Cemeteries and Crematoria Services, including the new head, Arnold, and was asked questions by a panel of four people – something I'd never experienced before in my life. I was terrified, even though they were all lovely. Thankfully, all that preparation paid off and I got the job. I left university with a Postgraduate Diploma and became a full-time trainee anatomical pathology technician. But just because I left university I knew I hadn't left behind my education. In fact, I was going to learn more, everything that was relevant to the path I wanted to take.

And thus began a new chapter of my life in death.

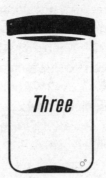

Three

Examination: 'Judging a Book by Its Cover'

As if you were on fire from within, the moon lives
in the lining of your skin.

—Pablo Neruda

I ran into the office one morning to find Andrew in his usual
seat, typing away. I could barely contain my glee.

'It's finally happened!' I squealed.

He looked up from his computer and frowned at me over
his spectacles.

'The day I've been waiting for!' I beckoned to him. 'Come
and have a look!'

Curious, he followed me into the fridge room. Once there, I
moved behind the trolley in the middle of the huge foyer with
my arms wide open, like a magician gesturing to an audience,

to give him a clearer view of the body bag and its contents: it was a man wearing very ordinary clothes and yet ... women's underwear. And not just any women's underwear: it was a whole pink lace ensemble, incredibly tight, that looked particularly uncomfortable over his nether regions as it mashed everything down. It was a surprise, not least because it didn't go with his rough countenance and facial hair as well as his tracksuit trousers and T-shirt, the former pulled down to his knees and the latter pulled up to his chin.

I mention this, not because I think cross-dressing is inherently funny, but because at that point – a year so into my training – I really felt like I'd been initiated into the world of mortuary work, having happened upon this unexpected cadaver. Every mortician has his share of unusual cases and this was to be one of many for me. But there's another reason I mention it. It's to illustrate that a post-mortem examination isn't just about removing organs and using fancy forensic techniques to determine what lies beneath; the examination begins with the outside of the body. In fact, usually as soon as the deceased is encountered in the mortuary. Sometimes external artefacts can be a clue to how and why a person died.

In most establishments, the fridges are opened and their contents checked against the mortuary registers first thing in the morning – a bit like doing a body stocktake after the overnight absence. Who knows what cases the police may have brought in from the streets in the middle of the night, or who may have been wheeled down from the wards? And the fridges, with their four or five shelves, can hold a lot of adults, their different scents merging to create a heady cocktail of death. In mortuaries with fewer staff you may need to book the new deceased in before or after you carry out the day's post-mortems, but if there are enough staff you may split the duties with some carrying out autopsies and others body-checking. Either way, it's an important part of the examination, and it takes two APTs if it's to be done properly so that they can vouch for each other.

Like gifts, the deceased should always be wrapped. Sometimes it will be in simple white cotton sheets, particularly when the patient has come from a hospital bed, and at other times it will be in body bags made of white plastic, or white plastic sheeting. From those very first days at the Municipal Mortuary right up to the end of my mortuary career I never considered the daily opening of the bags a chore. After each one was unzipped there was a pause and an atmosphere of suspense ... what might be inside? It always used to put me in mind of those Tonka toys called Keypers, from when I was a child. They were animals made from vibrant-coloured plastic and rubber, and their bodies opened up with a chunky key so you could store things inside, away from nosy younger siblings. One was a gorgeous pink swan and another was a peachy-coloured snail, but I had the majestic lilac horse and I adored it. It was the only one of my toys I never tried to do an autopsy on because she already opened up and I could see what was inside ... a tiny little surprise friend called a Finder!

As well as their surprise inside they had a very distinctive smell which, unfortunately, some of our body bags did too, but in a totally different way.

Suffice to say, to me every day was like Christmas Day in the mortuary. This was especially true one December when we opened a body bag to reveal a plump old man with white hair and beard in a full red jogging suit. To this day I'm not sure if he was purposely trying to resemble Santa or if it was just a huge coincidence.

Once the deceased is accessible, everything is noted in one glance: clothing, jewellery, money or wallet, medical intervention, visible tattoos, injuries and more. The height and weight of the deceased are written down for the pathologist and for the undertakers, who will be able to get a head start on the coffin order if they know the size in advance. This is done by using a long measuring stick and removing the patient's tray from the cold store on to the trolley which has scales attached, then pressing the button to manoeuvre them up and down with an electrical screech.*

Identity tags are then checked: there should be one on the wrist and one on the ankle, and they obviously need to match each other. Any jewellery the deceased is wearing is noted down if it hasn't already been recorded by the staff who delivered the body, and is double-checked by the APTs. There is a rule that the words 'gold' and 'silver' aren't used in mortuaries because we can't really be certain what metal items are actually made of. If we write 'gold ring' on the personal effects form and the next of kin see that and don't find a gold ring on their deceased – because it was just a yellow tin ring from Topshop, for example – they could sue us for a 'missing gold ring'. Instead, we say 'white metal' and 'yellow metal'. It's very festive when you get to sing 'Five yellow metal riiiiings!' to your colleague in the middle of December when logging property. For the same reason we never say 'diamond' or 'emerald' either – we say 'white stone' or 'green stone' instead.

---

* During a radio interview I once had a woman point out that her weight still being an issue *after* death was an irritating thought, and I can see her point.

Space can be at a premium in mortuary fridges – it's popular real estate; people are dying to get in there after all – so the turnaround from arriving in the facility and having a post-mortem, then being released, shouldn't be more than a couple of days. Often in the winter, when the death rate is higher, mortuary staff can descend into a bit of a panic if it looks as though the spaces are filling up, just in case there's some sort of mass fatality, or a spate of unrelated deaths due to the cold, and they run out of room.

'What are we supposed to do if the fridges get too full?' I panicked to Andrew that first winter I worked at the mortuary and saw the number of decedents we received increasing.

He explained to me that mortuaries may charge a rate to the Coroner if decedents are there too long without Coronial intervention and release; that is, ensuring they are moved to a funeral home or similar. 'It's a day rate,' he said. 'We call it B&B.'

'Well, really it's just "B",' I countered with a wink, and Andrew smiled. It was nice to see him not so serious for once.

So already, by simply encountering the deceased, the external examination has begun, and in addition to the information already garnered, visual cues add further pieces to the puzzle. The size of the deceased's body, whether excessively large or excessively slim, may have contributed to their death. Perhaps, in the case of anorexia or a wasting illness, the organs had simply failed? Obesity could indicate a heart attack, or else there may be visible injuries and external signs of what might have occurred. Another phenomenon noticeable on the exterior of the cadaver is evidence of one of forensic science's most well-known tenets, Locard's Exchange Principle, which stipulates that 'every contact leaves a trace'.

This guideline, attributed to French scientist Edmond Locard, dates from around 1910 and is the basic principle of all the 'trace evidence' referenced in crime fiction and on TV: hair and fibres, blood spatter and semen, footprints, tyre tracks and more. These can all be found at scenes, on the dead and on perpetrators, because every contact between one object and another causes materials from each surface to swap over. For our purposes, we can see from the body if the deceased had been involved in certain scenarios, particularly those to do with narcotics or violence. Leaves and twigs show someone was found dead outside, and conversely pen caps and newspaper print along with other household debris stuck to the decedent may indicate someone was discovered in an untidy home.

Immediately a picture begins to form.

The post-mortem colour of the deceased may also afford some sort of clue. People generally assume that all dead bodies are pale, but some are actually very pale: a dove grey compared to the usual ivory. It may take a while to notice these subtle differences but once you do you can diagnose a ruptured abdominal aortic aneurysm – or 'Triple A' – by how pale the deceased is, and how suddenly death occurred. This particular cause of death happens very quickly, when an aneurysm of the largest artery in the human body, the aorta, bursts. Blood gushes into the abdominal cavity, leaving the victim looking like the freshly bled victim of a vampire in a Hammer Horror film, giving us mortuary staff clues by sight.

Or perhaps the deceased is slightly pinker than would ordinarily be expected. This can indicate death by carbon monoxide (CO) poisoning, because the CO binds in an unusual way with the haemoglobin in the blood, giving the decedent a cherry-red tint. (Haemoglobin is the main oxygen-carrying compound in the blood, and its potential to do its job correctly is disrupted by the presence of CO.) Conversely, they may be blue, indicating cyanosis caused by inadequate oxygenation which points to completely different causes of death, such as asphyxiation. The vast rainbow of colours in which the patient may present keeps the APT guessing about the circumstances of death. Fluorescent yellow? Liver failure. Purple? Congestion. Green? Well, the less said about green the better, really.

Another important aspect of the preliminary examination of our fridge's residents is checking for pacemakers or implantable cardioverter defibrillators (ICDs), which are used to regulate people's heartbeat in life. These particular implanted devices must be removed if the patient is to be cremated because they can explode in the heat of the furnace. In fact, they tend to be removed anyway as they can be recycled, either whole or in part. (Whole, functioning pacemakers can be given to charities such as Pace4Life to be used in the developing world.) If the deceased has a post-mortem, then it's removed as part of that process, but if the person doesn't need a PM there is a way to remove it which is minimally invasive.

The first time I ever removed a pacemaker I was utterly convinced I'd kill myself. You see, pacemakers and ICDs are two different things and before any sort of incision can be made to remove them you must distinguish between the two.

Jason trained me for this. The procedure is classed as invasive, but it's probably the quickest and easiest to learn and therefore ideal for the trainee APT. One morning he handed me some gloves and a plastic apron and asked whether I was ready to 'tick something off that training and examination log'. The gloves and apron made me think I was in for yet more cleaning. Trainee APTs get pretty handy with a sponge, and at clearing sink drains of hairballs and yellow sludge, in their first few weeks of mortuary work. Although that sounds disgusting, it's actually incredibly important to ensure the drains don't get blocked with any remains, and using forceps to remove the debris can be satisfying and therapeutic. I used to go completely into a 'Zen' zone, pulling out globules and hair and leaving the plughole gleaming. That said, when Jason then went to retrieve some string, scissors and a scalpel, I happily guessed what was coming next. We had permission from the family to remove the pacemaker from the deceased and I had watched him carry out the procedure a couple of times. Now it was my turn.

I used my hands to feel for the device on the left side of the chest and could definitely discern its outline. They can be felt by palpating the skin, although that can be slightly more difficult if the patient is on the plump side as pacemakers are slim objects with rounded edges and the excess adipose tissue can obscure their gentle curves. Their purpose is to help control abnormal heart rhythms, or arrhythmias, with small electric pulses that encourage the heart to beat at a steady rate – not too fast or too slow but just right, which would please Goldilocks – so they need to be fairly innocuous and small.

As I hovered the scalpel blade over the flat front of the pacemaker I quickly looked up at Jason, alarmed. 'Are you sure it's not an ICD?'

An ICD is a larger device which can warn you of its

presence with its size, but I hadn't quite seen or felt enough of them to know the difference at that point. They're implanted into people who are at risk of a sudden cardiac arrest, and in the case of one occurring they administer massive electric shocks which kick-start the heart. These devices can't be removed like a normal pacemaker: if an unsuspecting APT cut through the wires with metal scissors it would give her a huge electric shock, possibly even kill her. Instead, the ICD pacing clinic has to be contacted so that a cardiac physiologist can attend and turn it off. They arrive with a small machine which they use to deactivate it and take readings, ensuring that the device is indeed no longer 'live'. It can then be removed in the same way as a pacemaker, although via a slightly larger incision, with no risk.

'I'm sure it's only a pacemaker, hun – but if it is an ICD at least you're wearing rubber shoes!' Jason said with a wink.

On this occasion, however, I didn't really have any nerves, despite it being my first ever incision into a human, because I only needed to make a slit around two inches long into the flesh. I knew I could handle *that* at least. Also, the person beneath my blade was not alive. As much as the deceased are still very much people to those who work in mortuaries, for me there is subconsciously a clear distinction between alive and dead. Later on, during my first full incision, I found that the phantom pain I'd felt with the anorexic dentist's bedsores was the one and only time it occurred and I'd quickly become immune to it. My brain seemed to grow to understand that the patient couldn't feel the scalpel and that I had a job to focus on and get done.

I made the short incision with the scalpel easily, right across the flat front of the pacemaker. Then, with a gloved thumb and forefinger on either side, squeezed the device up through it. The skin, yawning open to reveal yellow adipose tissue and the shiny surface of the pacemaker, put me in mind of a conker bursting out of its soft bed in a horse chestnut shell. The wires were still attached and I easily dealt with these by cutting them with the scissors. I then cleaned the device with disinfectant (our ever trusty Bioguard) and placed it into a labelled plastic bag to be collected at a later date by the Cardiac 'cath' lab. Finally I stitched up the small incision – I'd had some practice with this on Jason's previous pacemaker incisions – and it was barely noticeable. After I gently pressed a sticking plaster on top of the stitches and smoothed it down, the deceased was ready to be re-bagged.

'Well done, hun!' Jason said, as he ticked a box on my training log and signed his name next to it. I was one step closer to being a qualified APT.

Explosions in crematoria due to pacemakers were quite common before removals routinely took place, with the first reported incident happening in the UK in 1976. In fact, a 2002 paper in the *Journal of the Royal Society of Medicine* found that about half of all crematoria in the UK had experienced pacemaker explosions which caused structural damage and injury. The most recent was a case from the late 1990s in Grenoble, France, in which the pacemaker of a pensioner exploded with the force of two grams of TNT and caused around £40,000 worth of damage. The widow (who hadn't informed the crematorium of the pacemaker) and the doctor (who never checked for one) were both found liable for negligence and ordered to pay damages.

In addition to pacemakers and ICDs, there are other implants that need to be noted on examination and possibly removed if the deceased is to be cremated, so we had to really take notice of the body and the paperwork. During cursory external examinations one of the most obvious additions is breast implants, particularly in older ladies, as they stand to serious attention, defying gravity when everything else has nestled down into the tray. In fact, they are even more notice-able on the dead than on the living because they cool and stiffen so much in the fridge that they resemble two police helmets. However, they're not a huge problem in a furnace as they tend to just create a sticky residue that eventually burns up.

The same can't be said of a relatively new type of metal implant called Fixion Nails which are used to treat fractures of large bones, such as the humerus in the arm, and the tibia and femur in the leg. These expandable devices slide into the medullary cavity of the bone and are pumped up via a hydraulic mechanism filled with saline. In 2006, a published paper described the implications of this new device in the deceased when a seventy-nine-year-old man was cremated with one in his arm:

> At the crematorium, one of the staff was overseeing the firing of the oven through a transparent observation port when the coffin exploded. This was felt and heard by other staff elsewhere in the building. Extensive damage was caused to the oven, and considerable distress to the staff. It transpired that the cause of the explosion was the humeral nail.

Since the hydraulic Fixion Nail is filled with saline, the heat from the crematorium machine causes the salt water to expand into a gas which explodes in its tight metal casing.

This kind of story illustrates the importance of a good cursory external examination, keeping an eye open for every possibility. After these checks have been completed, the deceased can go back into the fridge while we await news as to whether or not they will require the full post-mortem examination.

Does *anyone* like examinations? Whether it's a dental exam, a breast exam or an academic exam, the word usually has a negative connotation. But we can't get away from examinations: we have them for everything – even, it seems, when we're dead.

In order to progress from my role as mortuary assistant or trainee APT I had to take an exam myself, in Anatomical Pathology Technology. This is usually taken after two years, a period during which the practical training log is also completed. I, however, took mine after one year due to previous experience in embalming as well as my work on my degree. There was then the option to progress from APT to Senior APT with another two years of work and examinations. Although this is as long as a degree, it's a technical qualification and not a medical one.* The difference between APTs

---

* Though this has actually now changed to a Level 3 and Level 4 Diploma.

and pathologists is that pathologists are qualified doctors who first complete a medical degree, then go on to specialise in pathology, which is the study of death and disease. They have a lot more exams and treat live people for many years first, something I absolutely didn't want to do: my fascination was with processes that occurred *after* death and how that could tell a story.

When I was working on the first part of the APT training process and aiming for the Certificate, I dreaded my examination portion. The actual learning, however, was fantastic, especially because it was literally hands on and I had the resources I needed. When being questioned about human anatomy by the pathologist or Jason I could see it there in front of me, and when attempting a certain incision I would watch it several times before trying it myself. I had a valid reason to be learning these skills – skills that would be for the greater good of society, helping to diagnose disease or assisting pathologists in forensic autopsies which could put murderers behind bars – and there were no real obstacles to me achieving that.

But imagine trying to obtain anatomical knowledge and learn invasive techniques with nothing to practise on. This has been an issue faced by medical students of many eras: how can you become a surgeon or doctor if you aren't familiar with the human body? In the absence of humans for dissection, what can be used? Artificial models? Animals? Perhaps, but only to a point. As the eminent English surgeon and anatomist Sir Astley Cooper said two centuries ago, 'He must mangle the living if he has not operated on the dead.'

Human dissection and examination for education has fallen in and out of favour over millennia depending on political and religious beliefs. The enlightened Ancient Greeks didn't consider dissection to be an immoral desecration of the dead: they thought of it as an extension of science's empirical nature. The Greek physicians Herophilus of Chalcedon and Erasistratus of Chios are therefore considered the first to have systematically dissected human cadavers and recorded their findings, in the third century BC, and they went on to found the great medical school in Alexandria. The problem, however, was that all that free rein may have made Herophilus a bit *too* enthusiastic: it has been said he actually vivisected – that's dissected *alive* – around six hundred prisoners. But with the advent of the Roman Empire, dissection became illegal anyway. This was due to religious beliefs: Roman law held that interference with a dead body was impious or blasphemous. This forced physicians like Galen of Pergamon, who was a follower of Herophilus, to dissect and examine Barbary apes and other animals in around AD 200, then apply that knowledge to humans. Galen suggested that we have two jawbones like a dog, but we don't. He also thought that blood passed from one side of the heart to the other via tiny holes, rather than the circulatory system we know about today. There were many inconsistencies in his work but this didn't stop Galen's 'knowledge' being uncontested for over 1300 years. Galen had done the best he could with limited means but without the correct resources much of his inference was purely speculation.

It was finally discovered to be guesswork with the advent of the Renaissance, when medical teaching began to flourish during a systematic growth in the sciences which continued over a few hundred years. As part of this more enlightened culture eighteenth-century Paris, for example, developed a system of donating cadavers to medical schools that was much more advanced than in the UK and US. But cadavers were still in short supply even for established institutions. The students' anatomy demonstration would consist of a learned professor instructing a barber-surgeon to carry out the dissection of a single corpse while they all observed. Their education was not quite 'hands on'.

If Galen could be considered the 'Mel Gibson' of anatomy and dissection (old has-been with some funny ideas) then the 'Ryan Gosling' (young upstart heart-throb) of the art would be Vesalius. Anatomist Andreas Vesalius, born 1514, was a child of the new era – a real rebel, but certainly one with a cause. He was also quite good-looking if etchings from the time are anything to go by. (Perhaps rosy-cheeked Renaissance ladies pasted these etchings of him on their bedroom walls and made euphemistic comments about *his* anatomy, who knows?) He was a determined and intelligent student who'd entered the University of Paris in order to fulfil a lifelong desire to be an anatomist, beginning in a childhood spent catching and dissecting small animals. At eighteen years old he was excelling in his studies and, eager to learn as much as he could, he would often sneak out to steal the recently executed cadavers from the notorious Gibbet of Montfaucon outside Paris's city walls, and examine skulls and bones in the Holy Innocents Cemetery. He'd return home silently with his precious quarry, and carry out his examinations of corpses in the dead of night, by candlelight. But this apparently sinister behaviour paid off: by the age of only twenty-two Vesalius was presenting his own anatomy lectures to budding students and dissecting the cadavers himself. His illustrated magnum opus *De Humani Corporis*

Fabrica ('On the Structure of the Human Body'), published in 1543, finally showed that Galen wasn't a reliable source of anatomical knowledge.

Like all revolutionaries, Vesalius had his detractors who refused to believe in the credibility of this young maverick and he was continually forced to justify himself. But for medical students and anatomists it was now clear that the old ideas could not be relied upon, and that dissection, which had been prohibited in Britain until the sixteenth century, was necessary for the advancement of their education. Soon they would stop at nothing to have the experience themselves.

In the UK, when formal universities began to teach young surgeons, the only cadavers legally donated to medical schools for examination were done so via the Murder Act of 1752. This meant that executed criminals would find themselves the star of the show on the stage of the dissection theatre, whether they wanted to or not. The Act's intention was twofold: it supplied research materials to desperate students, but it also acted as a deterrent for would-be criminals. It was one of many sadistic double-punishments in operation at the time, because back then death wasn't enough: the corpse itself had to suffer some form of abuse, which usually involved it being chopped into pieces. Examples include being hanged, drawn and quartered, or decapitated post-mortem and having your head thrust on to a stake like a marshmallow on a skewer. The rationale was simple: come Judgement Day, when the dead were to be raised from the Earth to stand before the gates of Heaven (according to the Bible), there was no chance of being let in if you were in four chunks, or missing parts of yourself and dripping all over the place like a leaky rubbish bag. Apparently, no one wanted Heaven to look like the waiting room in *Beetlejuice*. Being dissected was the Christian equivalent of not getting into the club because you aren't wearing a tie. The negative associations with human dissection, organ donation, plastination and even cremation that are still evident today are in part a hangover from that particular religious fear.

Despite the Murder Act, there were not enough cadavers for the nine or ten UK universities offering Medicine as a degree in the 1800s and the shortage led to the infamous trade of body snatching carried out by Resurrection Men. Just like Vesalius, the body snatchers would head to graveyards in the dead of night in search of freshly interred corpses. They were professionals who used wooden spades rather than metal ones so that the tell-tale clank of spade on soil couldn't be heard by passers-by. They opened the coffin at the head end, then tied a rope around the upper portion of the deceased and heaved them out with minimal disruption. All clothing and any jewellery had to go back into the coffin because there was a law against grave-robbing, but not body snatching – something the Resurrection Men were well aware of. It was a tightly run operation with one goal: to claim a body for dissection. The difference was that they weren't medical men themselves carrying out these acts to advance their own knowledge, they were just ordinary men in it for the money. These gangs were the go-betweens of the medical schools and the mausoleums, paid by those who ran the universities to retrieve as many viable corpses as possible for their students. And they were paid well – some earned a few months' average salary in just one week of body snatching – plus they had summers off: dissections, for refrigeration reasons, were only carried out in autumn and winter. In fact, some medical school students paid for their tuition with the revenue they made from body snatching; Ruth Richardson writes on the subject, 'in Scotland anatomy students could pay for their tuition in corpses rather than coin'.

St Bartholomew's Hospital, where I'm now based, was no stranger to the body trade once surgeon John Abernethy set up the successful medical school in around 1790.* The infamous Fortune of War pub stood right across from the hospital, although it was demolished in 1910, and there is just a monument there now. The inscription is very telling:

> The Fortune of War was
> The chief house of call
> North of the River for
> Resurrectionists in body
> snatching days years ago.
> The landlord used to show
> The room where on benches
> Round the walls the bodies
> Were placed labelled
> With the snatchers'
> names waiting till the
> Surgeons at Saint
> Bartholomew's could run
> Round and appraise them.

---

* Incidentally, he gives his name to the Abernethy Biscuit, a sweet baked snack which was created in 1829 to aid digestion. This is because he believed diseases were frequently the results of disordered states of the digestive organs, and were to be treated by purging and attention to diet – a theory still very popular today.

This engraving doesn't make it clear whether or not there was a separate room for the corpses, or if they were on benches in the main bar where all the ordinary workers were trying to wet their whistles. If the latter, I'm assuming it spurred a few of the punters to drink more than they normally would.

Many of the deterrents created to stop tradesmen from gaining access to fresh corpses were expensive and only the rich could afford them. These included paying guards to watch the grave night and day, mort-safes (iron cages placed over the grave that dug deep into the soil and protected the cadaver) and even cemetery guns to fire at those who would enter the graveyard under the cloak of night. Eventually, people started to grow tired of having to watch over their dead loved ones for days on end to ensure they weren't stolen and sold on. The final straw came with the case of Burke and Hare in Scotland. The pair had decided that digging up corpses was just too much effort and instead started simply to murder people and sell their (very fresh) merchandise to Dr Robert Knox, who taught anatomy at the Royal College of Surgeons of Edinburgh and was willing to turn a blind eye to their crimes (quite literally, as it happens: he was blind in one eye after contracting smallpox as a child). The subsequent outcry at these murderers' motives meant that the 'abhorrent trade in body snatching' was put to an end with the Anatomy Act of 1832 which ensured that, just as Paris had been doing for years, bodies of the unclaimed dead from hospitals and workhouses and from the streets could be donated to reputable schools.

Although it may seem like the history of anatomy is populated with the odd weirdo, in general it comprises upstanding scientific men who simply needed a way to learn and teach. It's the scarcity of cadavers which explains medical collections like the one I currently work with. These potted anatomical and pathological specimens were specifically removed from the few bodies available at the time, as well as some live patients during surgery, as a lasting testament and a teaching aid for many years to come. They were displayed in specialist medical collections for trainee surgeons, and even in museums, open to the public, complete with other 'oddities' like anatomical waxes and strange animal preparations. They eventually evolved into carnival sideshow attractions at the beginning of the twentieth century but their original use had been honourable and, even as a public spectacle, they still had the ability to teach as well as horrify. This meant that initially exhumations and dissections were not carried out in vain and as much good came from them as possible. In the years before my examinations for my mortuary work I also used specimens from similar collections, like the Hunterian Museum in London, in order to learn. They were hundreds of years old but still had the ability to teach anatomy and pathology to a modern-day APT. Now, as technical curator of the collection at Bart's, I feel like I've come full circle and I do what I can to impart that same knowledge to others.

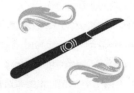

Most examinations aren't possible without a simple piece of paper, and the external exam of a corpse is no different. The typical 'external form' used in mortuaries is fairly similar all over the world and has two images on it: one is a naked, bald, asexual figure from the front, and the other is the same but from the back.

These universal representations of the human form are to be populated by little symbols that correspond to any external features witnessed on the deceased once they've been undressed. You can simply put a big 'X' in the relevant place to demarcate a tattoo or an injury, for example, but I liked to draw tiny versions of tattoos, birthmarks and scars on my forms, in part for realism and in part just because it helped me bestow the case with a true identity.

As with much else, it was Jason who first introduced me to these external forms, but after a while he left the Municipal Mortuary and moved on to one at a hospital five minutes away from ours. He was replaced by June, another locum from Liverpool, who would oversee the rest of my training. It was fantastic to have someone new to learn from and particularly refreshing for that person to be a woman. It was the beginning of a real shift in the gender of mortuary workers, when women seemed to start entering the ranks. Interestingly, it wasn't actually a first for women. In nineteenth-century Germany, so-called Waiting Mortuaries employed the very first attendants of the dead: females called *leichenfraus* ('corpse brides') who laid out the deceased, tended to their appearance and made funeral arrangements. Then, once those Dead Houses were established in England, the deceased would be 'guarded and watched day and night by a resident attendant. The appointment of a woman as the first keeper and the purchase by the burial board of a "suitable black dress" for her to wear, would have helped to reassure the public that the bodies of their family members would have been treated with care and dignity.'*

Since then we'd been through two world wars, but times were changing. Women were beginning to enter all sorts of previously male-oriented careers including the death industries, and June had been one of the first, having trained as an embalmer from the age of only sixteen as part of a Youth Training Scheme – a vocational training course for those who wanted to leave school at sixteen or seventeen. She had seen everything and, as well as having a lot to teach me, she was utterly hilarious.

One of the first patients June and I autopsied together was a harrowing case of a man who'd jumped from the top of a building, and by the time he was brought into the mortuary he was in several pieces. Over the two years or so I had been working in the mortuary I had seen many disturbing cases, from road traffic collisions to suicides, but this was one of the most fragmented. That so much damage could be inflicted on what I knew to be a sturdy frame left me curious but shaken. The human instinct is to both turn away and look at the same time – a natural oxymoron. The sight left me stunned. The left side of his skull had been completely crushed and this injury, along with his torn limbs and bones bursting through his flesh, rendered the external examination pretty difficult. I had to depict huge Frankenstein's monster-like stitches across the limbs on the external form to demarcate where they had been torn off. Some of his brains had been scooped up from the ground, deposited into a small plastic bag and brought to us along with his body.

---

* This from my favourite paper, the Pam Fisher one . . .

I'll never forget June's casual question to me: 'Did you find his left eyeball in that bag of brains?'

'Er, I haven't looked yet,' I'd answered nervously. Still trying to wrap my head around this difficult case, I hadn't got to the point of sifting through the soft grey matter for an eyeball that I wasn't yet sure was missing.

'Oh – it's OK, here it is,' June said, pointing to his right calf. The eyeball had somehow rolled underneath him and was poking out and staring up at us like a salmon's eye from a fishmonger's counter.

She took the clipboard from me and drew an eyeball poking out of the leg on the external form. She even gave it eyelashes and a little optical nerve. I laughed out loud but it turned into a sob – a sob I could just about hide with the laughter. I knew June was being facetious for a reason. She needed to take me out of my head for a second before I lost it. With that eyeball drawing she enabled me to spill out a bit of the emotion that might have hindered my work on the case. I felt relieved after that, as if I'd sneezed to clear my head, and could focus on the task at hand once again.

I took the clipboard back from her and continued cataloguing the severe injuries before me, all the while thinking I'd come a very long way from those days at university labelling dry bones on the page with technical terms like 'tibia' and 'calcaneus' and 'spheno-occipital synchondrosis'. As I'd guessed, the lectures and the textbooks just don't prepare you for the reality of the mortuary.

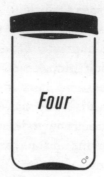

Difficult and Decomposed Examinations: 'Pulp Fiction'

Decline is also a form of voluptuousness.
Autumn is just as sensual as springtime. There
is as much greatness in dying as in procreation.
                                          —Iwan Goll

The scent of decomposition is formulated of molecules so meaty and musky it almost becomes corporeal. It nudges the back of your throat with an insistent, demented sweetness which feels as though you're being kissed far too deeply by a rotting tongue. But unlike TV programmes where rookie cops and jaded detectives alike shove menthol cream up their nostrils to mask the odour, APTs and pathologists have to learn to live with it. This is because all decomposing patients smell different, and in some of those dark olfactory rainbows there are clues as to how the deceased passed away – sometimes absolutely vital ones in a case where the organs have decayed into pulp and show no discernible pathologies. But in addition to this it's simply better to surrender yourself to the odours because eventually the brain stops receiving strong olfactory signals (like when you're convinced you can't smell the perfume you applied earlier but everyone else definitely can) and the smell becomes bearable, even comfortable.

I mentioned that, for the most part, unzipping the new body bags in the morning was a fairly positive experience for APTs who welcomed the opportunity to use their skills on a diverse range of cases. But there is something an APT may dread and it's not the distinctive and lovely powdery smell of Keypers, it's that ominous, cloying scent of a decaying corpse. It's implied as soon as you walk into the mortuary in the morning and get a whiff of the unmistakable odour, and it's confirmed when the deceased is pulled out of the fridge in a black body bag. A dramatic orchestral 'dun-dun-duuun' may as well erupt, followed by a cymbal crash and a lightning flash. The dreaded black body bags were much more hard-wearing than the thinner white bags, so among other things they were mainly used for what we called 'decomps' for short. If a black bag wasn't available then the deceased was double-bagged in the ordinary white ones – sometimes even *triple*-bagged – which was just as ominous for the APT. When staff opened the bag's zip to reveal yet more white plastic and another zip, it was like a game of pass the parcel they didn't want to play.

This industrial-strength wrapping was necessary to keep

a variety of things inside the bag and away from the other patients in the same fridge: smells, fluids, maggots, flies, snips, snails, puppy dog tails ... all the things that a decomp is made of.

I had a deal with June that she would carry out autopsies on all the bariatric bodies (which is the politically correct term for 'obese') if I did all the decomps. She was only too happy to oblige, although she couldn't understand my choice. 'Why? Why would you want that? What goes on in that head of yours, Tiny?' She called me Tiny because I was still hitting the gym hard and was very slim at the time – something that caused me some difficulty with the larger bodies. I explained this fear to her – the fear that I might fall into the body cavity, my legs comically poking out and flailing around.

Most APTs hate decomps with a passion but I didn't mind them; after all, I was a veteran due to my childhood spent directing funerals for roadkill. I found the decomposing deceased intriguing, and quickly became immune to the moist, squelchy noises, fetid smells and endless parade of insects. All these colonising creatures fascinated me, as did the topic of Forensic Entomology, which I'd studied at university, so I often collected maggots and other insects from autopsies in white-lidded Sterilin pots and conveyed them down the road to the World Museum, Liverpool, during my lunch break. I could happily chat to an entomologist about what species it was at the same time as eating my sandwich. They were always just the usual larvae and flies you'd expect to find in the UK – blowflies, cheese skippers, bluebottles – but I liked being there, talking entomology and looking through the myriad drawers of insects pinned down in their little white death-beds. The staff even came to know me as

'Maggot Girl' – a term of endearment, I assumed, although very descriptive of me in general: you see, I often needed to remove maggots from my clothing during autopsies, and once even from my bra.

It was unusual.

The maggots themselves weren't unusual, just the fact that they had managed to access my bra. Maggots are a weekly occurrence in some mortuaries and can be practically a daily one during the summer months. It's an unfortunate fact of life that many people, by choice or circumstance, die alone and aren't discovered for a long time. (Take the incredibly sad, albeit exceptional, case of Joyce Carol Vincent, found dead at home in 2006, although it was believed she had died in 2003. The TV was still on after three years.) This means that their cadavers become fair game for scavenging creatures either as a place to inhabit, a food source, or both.

Normally during a particularly messy autopsy I'd be wearing full PPE which includes a green cotton surgical gown over my scrubs.* As this isn't waterproof and is liable to soak up any errant fluids I could inadvertently lean into, a disposable plastic apron goes over that. A similar principle lies behind the use of white plastic sleeve protectors, because even though latex gloves cover the hands, they will only pull up as far as your wrists. The disposable sleeve protectors – elasticated at both ends and similar to futuristic shiny legwarmers – shield the absorbent gown sleeves from a possible creeping wave of blood and fluids which may silently ascend to the elbow. And it wasn't just the one

---

* We changed into new scrubs every day, throwing the old ones into the laundry for the hospital linen services to collect, wash and redeliver. Sometimes after decomps we'd remove them, shower and wear new ones.

pair of latex gloves I'd wear but two, with 'cut proof' fabric gloves worn between the layers like a safety sandwich. This is imperative to ward against possible scalpel or needle-stick injuries which are a daily danger during autopsies. We call these 'cut proof' fabric gloves 'chainmail' because they're woven through with an incredibly fine metal mesh to stop an errant blade from slicing through to the skin. However, the threads have to be relatively wide apart to allow for manual dexterity, which means that needle points, and even the tip of a scalpel, can sometimes prick through between them. This is where the extra latex comes in: the two layers 'wipe' away blood and debris at a microscopic level as the sharp metal penetrates, so even if it pierces skin there is marginally less chance of catching something. When it comes to trying not to catch communicable diseases, every little helps.

Add to this ensemble a hair net and plastic face visor which steams up with every breath, and you can imagine how hot and sweaty it can get carrying out an autopsy in the summer, and how 'glamorous' it looks.

This is why a maggot got into my bra: it was seriously sweltering in the tiny post-mortem room that day. The air-conditioning wasn't working, and not for the first time. More importantly, neither was the downdraft system which is specifically meant to force any airborne pathogens away from our faces and down to the floor where they can wreak less havoc. I'd decided to forgo the cotton gown and instead wear a plastic apron directly against my scrubs, and the plastic sleeve protectors against the skin of my arms. It seemed smarter than wearing the cotton gown as well and fainting with heat exhaustion halfway through the procedure, perhaps cracking my head on the corner of the PM table on my journey down.

I was between a rock and a hard place here.

However, I could still feel the suffocating effect of the plastic on my flesh as beads of sweat, with nowhere to go inside their impermeable prisons, simply rolled up and down, up and down, as my arms changed position. I also couldn't see through the visor which kept steaming up from the heat of my face, so I removed that too. Without a visor or surgical mask I did feel slightly more comfortable, but, wearing a hair net and holding a ladle to remove liquid fat and blood from the cavity, I looked like a demonic dinner lady.

'How are you doing over there, Tiny?' June called to me, a look of bemused humour on her face. She always thought I'd regret my decision to take the decomps, but I never did.

'I'm fine, I've got it. It's not so bad,' I responded, but then I felt something cold and wriggly drop through the 'V' of my scrubs top. With no gown to protect my décolletage I was wide open to this invasion. By the time the maggot had landed skilfully between the fabric of my bra and my breast I had dropped my PM40* and was frantically shaking the front of my scrubs and hopping from one foot to the other until I'd secured its release and it landed on the PM room floor. It was only then I realised June was doubled over with laughter – she'd seen it on my shoulder and had predicted the outcome without warning me. I plotted a way to get her back, and soon.

*

---

* Interestingly, we are taught to ignore our natural reflexes in the PM room and if we drop something to allow it to fall. This is because trying to catch a PM40 or brain knife in mid-air could result in the loss of several fingers. It's a strange thing to get used to.

Putrefying cadavers teeming with scavengers are an eco-system unto themselves. I don't really believe in literal reincarnation – that a person's mind and soul remain intact and inhabit different bodies or vessels over time – but looking at the activity of new-born larvae and scuttling beetles as they devoured decomposing flesh gave me an understanding of what the 'circle of life' really meant, and it was nothing to do with cartoon lions and cheesy Elton John songs. The First Law of Thermodynamics states that energy cannot be created or destroyed, it can only change form. This means that though the force can flow from one place to another, the total energy of an isolated system does not change. If we consider the Earth and all its flora and fauna an isolated system, then the vital force of all those who pass away must in turn animate the insects who feed on them or leach into the soil in which they are buried. The fruit and vegetables that feed us, as well as feeding the animals we eat, grow in that soil and in that way the energy is 'reincarnated' or changes form. Edvard Munch put it succinctly: 'From my rotting body, flowers shall grow and I am in them and that is eternity.'

But why is the decomposing cadaver such an ecosystem, or biome? It's necessary to explore the processes of decay in detail to establish why something seemingly so revolting sustains millions of creatures, and understand that without those creatures we'd be knee deep in corpses. If you're the kind of person who can't watch gruesome horror scenes in films, or jumps when a spider or rat appears, then you might want to skip this next section . . .

Decay starts when the heart stops, although of course many would argue that the Placebo song 'Teenage Angst' is more accurate with its lyric 'since I was born I started to decay'. However, for our purposes decomposition, often split into five stages – fresh, bloat, active decay, advanced decay and dry remains – begins immediately after death. We'll begin with 'fresh' – and I discovered early on that 'fresh' is a very relative term when associated with corpses. It doesn't mean fresh like fresh air; more fresh as in a freshly soiled nappy or fresh sewage; fresh as in 'OK, you're not going to want to put your face in this, but believe me, it could be *way* worse'.

Fresh

 During this stage, one of the most well-known indicators of death, post-mortem rigidity or rigor mortis, begins between one and four hours after death. It occurs because several proteins in the muscles, which 'join hands' to create movement in life, are unable to let go since the substance that would enable them to do so, adenosine triphosphate, isn't being formed any more. Rigor starts in smaller muscles such as those found in the eyelids, jaw, neck and fingers. Some of these small muscles are in the iris, which is why a test for death is to shine light into the eye: dead pupils won't react to the light by constricting. Others affected are the arrector pili, tiny muscles that move the hair of mammals, for example, to create goosebumps; it's this action, their making the hairs stand on end, which gave rise to the fallacy that the hair grows after death.* Between

---

* It's also due to dehydration and the skin shrinking back, which is what makes the fingernails look as though they grow too. They don't, of course.

four and six hours after death, larger muscles are affected by rigor and the first stage of flaccidity (primary flaccidity) is over as the body becomes stiff and immobile. Rigor takes such hold of the limbs that attempting to move them into a different position can actually break the joints. I've heard the loud crack of this myself, although I've never been strong enough actually to break rigor, and I've never had reason to.

Most of the cases I've autopsied have been in one stage of rigor or another, and sometimes this can hinder the examination. For example, during the external exam, the pathologist must examine the genitalia and anus – it's part of a sequenced process that is the same for every single body so that nothing is missed. In some women's cases the pathologist and I have had to take a stiff leg each and heave them apart slowly, like pulling giant levers, to gain access. It's not dignified, no, but the checks are done in every autopsy so the pathologist can report any disease or ensure there's been no sexual violation. If there has been and it's not detected, it could mean the perpetrator walking free.

Much of what happens in a post-mortem examination may look undignified, but it's all an essential part of the process. Even so, there are times when I've been over-sensitive and the touch or actions of a pathologist have alarmed me. In one case, I remember a homeless pregnant girl, only fifteen years old, had committed suicide by jumping from a building. Her last known address was a care home and she had a severe drugs problem. Suicide, drugs, pregnancy and homelessness: all this at just fifteen. The pathologist I was with on the case had a group of medical students in the room with us and I understood they were there to learn. She had genital warts, the teenager, and when the doctor noticed and asked me to help spread her legs, which were in rigor, to show the students I just snapped and screamed 'No!' I couldn't help but think about how this girl had already been failed so many times, had probably been unable to protect herself, had likely suffered many indignities and violations. I couldn't let her suffer yet another; I couldn't just allow all these students to peer at her private parts like she was some specimen when they could easily see genital warts on a consenting live patient. They weren't pertinent to this case. The pathologist looked at me and didn't say anything about my outburst. I think he could tell by the look in my eyes that it was just unnecessary this time.

 Around the time the body has fully succumbed to rigor mortis, another indicator of death becomes more obvious. This is hypostasis, also called lividity or livor mortis (both Latin for 'purple' or 'bluish'). The reason we say someone is livid when they're angry is because their face goes purple. Lividity is a purpley-pink staining of the skin caused when the blood stops flowing and sinks downwards due to gravity. This means it settles or pools in the vessels at the points lowest down, except in those parts that are in contact with something, because those vessels are constricted or pressed closed. So if a person died lying on her back, for example, her upper back and shoulder blades would be white where they were in contact with the bed. Her buttocks, calves and heels would also remain white, or blanched. Any tight clothing, like bra straps, could cause blanching too. Sometimes in cases I worked on this was so clear that I could read the impression of the brand name around people's waists: Calvin Klein or Superdry.

At around ten hours this discolouration becomes very prominent, and can become what is known as 'fixed' after about twelve – this means the difference in skin tone, dark lividity and paler blanching, will not change back. It's a variable process so isn't always a good indicator of exact time of death, but if a cadaver is moved before fixation – say, from a chair to a bed – a second pattern will form and investigators can use this to indicate if someone is lying about how that body was found. In my experience, all sorts of things make patterns in the skin, and can reveal a lot about the death scene. Hypostasis happens whatever position the deceased is in so a person who hanged himself will have a much paler torso but his legs will be so full of blood they'll turn dark purple. This is called 'congestion'. Congestion is one of the reasons it may seem like a hanged man has died with an erection, but in reality the pooling blood is just flowing into every nook or cranny it can due to gravity.

It's very important that a pathologist and an APT can distinguish between hypostasis and bruising during the external examination, as genuine bruises may indicate the circumstances which led to someone's death. They can have very particular patterns which help to give us information. For example, bruised shins are common in alcoholics who frequently stumble around and bang into their furniture at home. Taken with other evidence such as liver disease and the sickly sweet smell of alcohol in the blood (another reason we don't shove menthol up our noses), we begin to tease out the story of how the decedent passed away.

During one of our cases – a lady who was a known alcoholic – the pathologist became suspicious of a set of bruises on the woman's upper arm.

'What do these look like to you?' he asked me.

'Finger marks,' I replied, corroborating his thoughts.

There was a distinct set of four elliptical bruises in a line down her tricep, as though someone had grabbed her upper arm with their hand. Taken with all the other injuries on her, it now looked like she could have been beaten rather than just stumbled around and injured herself. At the same time, there was marked hypostasis changing the colour of huge portions of her skin. The pathologist decided it was better to be safe than sorry and halted the Coronial post-mortem to refer it back to the Coroner, who would have to order a forensic post-mortem. We had to be absolutely sure that this woman hadn't been a victim of manslaughter or murder and a forensic PM is a different procedure, usually carried out by a different doctor, one trained not just in pathology but forensic pathology.

Another pet peeve here: forensic comes from the Latin *forensis* which means 'before the forum', such as a jury. It means something pertaining to the law. So on TV when a documentary says, for example, an Egyptian mummy is going to be 'forensically examined', it's not ... unless the mummy is a victim of crime or stands accused of a crime.* What they are using are analytical techniques which are sometimes applied forensically, in a criminal case. Forensic PMs require completely different staff to be in attendance: investigating police officers as well as exhibits officers and a photographer, in case the evidence needs to be presented in court. That's why a routine Coronial PM can't just become a

---

* Unbelievably, something like this *has* happened before. Pope Formosus was exhumed from his grave in Rome in AD 897 and put on trial in what became known as the Cadaver Synod (or, more appropriately, *Synodus Horrenda*).

forensic one – it's a whole different procedure. New paper-work has to be started from scratch and often a new venue and pathologist found.

The deceased is also by now quite cold, having suc-cumbed to another indicator of death: algor mortis, or post-mortem cooling. A sweeping generalisation is that the dead body loses 2°C in the first hour after death then 1°C per hour thereafter, until ambient temperature is reached. Again, there are many factors that may affect this, such as a fever, which would give someone a higher temperature at death and delay cooling. For the most part, the autopsies I've carried out have been on cold flesh, which is also relatively stiff because the deceased will have been in the mortuary fridge and human fat, just like butter, solidifies as it cools. But on the odd occasion a patient may come down from the wards and require an immediate PM – while still warm. Some people who work with the dead hate this as it's just too human; too real. It feels more like surgery and less like an autopsy. I never minded the warmth. Despite all those layers of gloves I was sensitive to the cold and it would make my fingers stiff, so the warmth was a bit of a relief for me. (Being a mortician has some odd perks, but you take them where you can get them.)

Between thirty-six and forty-eight hours after death, those 'hand-holding' proteins which caused rigidity have started to degrade, so rigor mortis finally loses its grip. This leads to secondary flaccidity, and the body won't stiffen again. The reason these proteins have degraded is that decomposition proper has started to become noticeable, and this can be split into two distinct pathways: autolysis and putrefaction.

Autolysis is believed to start four minutes after death. It means self-digestion and comes from the Greek *auto* meaning 'self' and *lysis* meaning 'split' or 'separation'. (That's why 'electrolysis' in beauty clinics means 'the separation of the hair from the body, using electricity'.) It's *self*-digestion because the intrinsic enzymes we have in our cells, normally useful for breaking down unwanted molecules, are released after death. They roam unchecked in the body, like rioters aware of a sudden lack of a police presence, who can't control the path of their own destruction once they've begun. One particularly self-destructive organ, the pancreas – responsible for producing the enzymes that help us digest food – simply digests itself. This is 'abiotic' decomposition (meaning 'without life' – a breakdown caused by chemical processes). It leads to an imbalance in the cells' structures and an increase in fluids which can cause blisters full of red or brown fluid to bloom on the skin; their eventual bursting causes skin sloughage, or 'skin-slip', about a week or so after death. It's this sloughage that enables us to remove the skin of the decomp's hand, like a glove, and wear it over our own latex to fingerprint the dead, if necessary. It can make tattoos and bruising, which are naturally positioned in the deeper layers of the skin, much more visible – so we tend to use a damp sponge to wipe off this layer, which comes away like stocking fabric. The blisters, heavy with dark red fluid, burst at the slightest touch or movement of the body anyway, hence the need for the industrial-strength wrapping in the fridge before PM.

Bloat

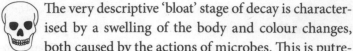 The very descriptive 'bloat' stage of decay is character-
ised by a swelling of the body and colour changes,
both caused by the actions of microbes. This is putrefaction. Where autolysis is abiotic, putrefaction is simply
biotic, relying on the activity of microbes in the body: living
helpers and not enzymes. These microbes are always present
in humans during life but, due to the effects of autolysis and
the subsequent breakdown of cells, they are able to invade the
usually prohibited parts of the living host, and, to top it off,
they are also suddenly awash with nutrient-rich fluids, so
they basically go 'on a bender'. The gastric population does
include fungi but the majority is the 'normal flora' of the gut
such as the genera Lactobacilli and Clostridia (one is the
helpfully named *Clostridium cadaveris* so there's no doubt as
to when it's this particular bacterium's time to shine). We're
all far more aware of our friendly bacteria now thanks to
Multibionta and Yakult adverts on TV, and it's worth remembering that the more of this flora you have in your system, the
quicker you'll putrefy when the time comes. That's one to
remember when you are encouraged to take the Actimel
challenge!

Although putrefaction occurs just after death, it takes a few
days for the signs to become noticeable. The bacteria cause
the colour fluctuations in the skin from green to purple to
black because haemoglobin, which gives blood its red colour,
is changed to sulphaemoglobin, a different substance containing infamously smelly sulphur. Because of their start
position in the gut, the first obvious sign of decay is usually a
greenish patch in the lower right of the abdomen (above the

caecum) which eventually moves across the belly and over the rest of the body. This green patch is such an irrevocable indication of decomposition it's one of the reasons those Dead Houses and Waiting Mortuaries were created in the 1800s. As Dr Maze pointed out in Quigley's *The Corpse: A History*, 'The only sure sign of death is putrefaction.' As well as protecting the living from the dead, there was the added benefit of the dead not being buried until this was witnessed, thus ensuring they weren't buried alive.

Soon, the effect of putrefaction can be very clearly seen across the shoulders and thighs as marbling, caused by the pigment from the colour-changing microbes taking the path of least resistance through the veins – at first, anyway. Eventually, the vessels also disintegrate and the bacteria roam even more freely. Gases build up in the tissues from the actions of all the bacteria, particularly *Clostridium perfringens*, which also causes the delightful-sounding 'gas gangrene' in the living. *C. perfringens* produces what mortuary-types call 'tissue gas'; it's this gas that makes a crackling or popping sound, called crepitation, when the cadaver is handled, as the flesh has become aerated just like a chocolate Aero (although much less palatable). The gas has very few places to go so it builds up in the cells. It sometimes escapes via the intestine as a post-mortem fart or through the mouth as a burp or groan (both indescribably smelly), but for the most part the collapse of the various natural exit tubes means the deceased begins to swell to an unnatural size. Without an escape route the tongue and eyes protrude, the genitals become engorged and the abdomen reaches what can only be described as 'bovine' proportions due to the increase in internal pressure.

I discovered the presence of this gas the hard way during my first ever decomp autopsy, when my boss, Andrew, watched me bend over the deceased, right over the top of the body, so I could see what I was doing. I took my PM40 and confidently made the incision as I normally would, yet when the blade breached the skin of the distended abdomen the green, taut flesh rippled and burst like a balloon from hell and I was rewarded with a face full of the most hideous gas I'd ever smelled in my entire life. I was wearing a face shield but it was no match for this eruption. To give you an idea of how it smelled, let's first consider the names of these gases: putrescine and cadaverine, created when proteins break down. Then there's hydrogen sulfide (rotten eggs) and methane (farts). There's also a compound called Skatole which I think would be more honestly represented if it were pronounced 'scat-hole', since 'skato' and therefore 'scat' are derived from the Greek meaning dung. I turned to Andrew, eyes narrowed behind a visor splattered in yellow and green globules, with a look that said *Why didn't you warn me?* To which he laughed and replied, 'Well, you'll never forget to stand back in future.'

Lesson well and truly learned, sir, and that's the reason I'm now reluctant to remove my face visor, despite the discomfort . . .

Piercing the abdomen at post-mortem offers this putrid gas an escape route, but in the absence of that a body may well continue to swell, forcing fluids out through orifices, becoming larger and larger until it actually bursts – by now perhaps a fortnight or so after death. And, yes, it may seem unbelievable but we do still need to carry out a full autopsy: the organs all need to be removed and inspected, which is not easy when they have totally lost their structural integrity. They go from being fairly distinct shapes of a very soft consistency to literally becoming a pulp. At this point everything is a pulp: organs, fat, liquid oozing from blisters. I'd try to remove the organs and they'd just run through my fingers like molasses.

One of the most interesting aspects of this decomposition stage is how totally unrecognisable it makes the cadaver, obscuring the person's real size, race, hair colour and facial features, sometimes even gender. In a small city like Liverpool, many deaths would be reported in the local newspaper as obituaries, with accompanying pictures of the deceased while they were alive. When working on a decomp case I'd build up a mental image of the patient only to find out later they looked nothing like I imagined, and it's this that taught me early on that visible identification of a decomposed decedent by family or friend is frequently not reliable enough.

Active Decay

This is the period of greatest mass loss because excess fluid will have been purged and gases will have left the body by some means (perhaps a wet-behind-the-ears autopsy technician with a sadistic manager swallowed most of it, who knows?).

The mass of the cadaver also decreases, meaning much of the body's flesh is consumed, because of the insatiable scavenging action of many creatures, among them my old friend, the maggot. As revolting as they may seem, flies and their larvae – maggots – are created perfectly for the job they need to do and many experts call them 'the unseen undertakers of the world'. Those oviparous flies which lay their eggs on the dead, and which I referred to earlier as the sort you'd expect to find in the UK, are mainly bluebottles from the *Calliphora* genus, which have a very reliable scavenging schedule. They lay eggs on orifices or wounds only, because the very young larvae need to eat decaying flesh but can't break the skin to feed. These flies arrive on the scene within twenty-four hours – as though they have a flash-mob Facebook group and receive notifications – depositing eggs which then hatch the next day. Another type of fly has a slight advantage in that it's viviparous and doesn't lay eggs but tiny maggots, which can start consuming flesh immediately. These are descriptively named *Sarcophagidae* or 'flesh flies'.*

Hundreds of these tiny larvae feed and feed, increasing in size through three different stages, or 'instars', at the rate of one every twenty-four hours. By the time they've reached their largest size, or third instar, they are a writhing mass of plump white 'rice'. Their feeding frenzy produces so much energy it can warm the cadaver by up to 50°C, and the maggots in the centre which overheat gradually migrate to the outside of the pulsing mass to cool down and allow others to access the middle in white rippling waves. They dive head-first into their nutrient-rich banquet, so dedicated to feeding they've developed hooks on their heads to keep them attached

---

* In case you'd like to learn yet more languages, *sarco* comes from the Greek for 'flesh' and *phage* means 'eat'. A sarcophagus is so named because people believed placing their dead in stone coffins helped the flesh to be consumed. And if anything, at least you now know it helps to be multi-lingual when studying decomposition.

to the slippery surface, moist from the enzymes they secrete to dissolve the flesh in order to slurp it. The two little dots at the other end, which look like they could be tiny black eyes, are actually spiracles, used to breathe out of their backsides. They are perfect little feeding machines which don't need to stop and come up for air, which is why they can consume 60 per cent of a human body in one week. When they are finally sated, they slink away slowly for a lie-down, much like we do after a huge meal; but the difference is they pupate, as when caterpillars become chrysalises, whereas we just put the TV on and fall into a carb-coma.

When working on decomp cases those wriggling maggots ended up everywhere: in my hair, inside my steel-toed boots, caught in the folds of my clothes and, of course, in my bra. And I couldn't simply brush them up and put them in a bin because they'd still pupate and the pupae are very resilient, like hard little nuts. There was only one way to deal with them: using the vacuum attachment of our head saw, I'd hoover them all up into a clean bag; then I'd put it on the PM room floor and jump up and down on it. It was very therapeutic, like pressing bubble wrap: I'd hear each one pop under my heavy boots until, a bit like popcorn in the microwave, the sound became less and less frequent so I knew I'd popped most of them. Then I'd throw the whole thing in an incineration bag with a tight cable tie and put it in the incinerator waste.

Maggot Girl turned on her own people.

Advanced Decay

This fourth stage of decay is loosely begun when the last of the satisfied maggots has rolled off the corpse and slithered off into a dark crevice to wait for its pupa to form. This can be up to fifty metres away, a huge distance for a creature which is only a centimetre long (that equates to a distance of about five kilometres for humans). During this phase the mass of the cadaver will have decreased considerably, which is why we are not knee deep in corpses; but the fluids created by the actions of autolysis and putrefaction will be evident in the surrounding floor, whether it's wood, carpet or soil.

The maggot is now quite resilient, having somehow avoided 'trial by hoover and boot', encased in a hard material inside which it will remain for ten to twenty days – and let's face it, after that ordeal it deserves a long rest. Any escapees will eventually emerge as cocky flies but without much time to show off: they'll start buzzing around the PM room then hit the strategically placed 'Insectocutors' and die in tiny sparks of glory, making the blue light flash on and off as if it were at a disco.

Maggots' association with the dead is well established but increasingly the general public has become aware of their use on the living. Maggot therapy is a form of treatment used for debriding necrotic tissue from wounds – basically removing dead tissue and leaving the healthy tissue alone. Even though the practice has been known of since antiquity it was more popular pre-antibiotics – around the 1930s – but has become so again since the medical world realised some microbes were becoming resistant to antibiotics, for example MRSA (Methicillin-resistant *Staphylococcus aureus*). On battlefields it was noticed that maggots would colonise the wounds of some soldiers and in those instances the injuries were less likely to be fatal; ostensibly, the maggots were eating away the infection and cleaning the wounds better than any other method known to physicians at the time, ensuring in the process that the wounded soldiers were spared from the blood poisoning which our anorexic dentist had succumbed to. Their use for this type of debridement is much lauded today and they are seen as beneficial, if a little gruesome.

But there is something maggots may be less well known for and that is the infestation of living creatures, including humans – a phenomenon known as myiasis. During our external examinations, as well as checking for bruises, tattoos and other artefacts both ante- and post-mortem, it's imperative that we raise the deceased onto their side and inspect the back. Imagine forgetting to do this, puzzling over how on earth a person died, then flipping them over to discover a huge shotgun wound between the shoulder blades! The full examination, carried out in the same front-and-back sequence each time, ensures this doesn't happen. What I was never prepared for were those unfortunate, neglected souls who had suffered from myiasis. It can occur in vulnerable humans who have been mistreated, for example children still in the same filthy nappy they've had on for weeks because of negligent parents, or old people left in one position to defecate on their bed and form bedsores, which subsequently become infected by their excrement, which is why it's frequently found on the posterior surface. It's an unnatural infestation, a consequence of man's heinous inhumanity to man, and something which once seen can never be forgotten.

So I feel justified in my enthusiasm for the natural ecosystem of a decaying corpse and the creatures that contribute to a sacred cycle of life. To me it's better than pondering those other actions which are most inhuman and unnatural.

Dry Remains

 Finally, we come to a relatively more manageable stage of decomposition, which is classed as 'dry remains' because only bones, cartilage and toughened skin are left. This category can include the familiar sights of bog bodies in museums and Egyptian mummification. The Egyptians may have called it 'embalming' but unlike modern embalming it was really just a way to dry out and preserve the remains, with each step having a profound religious significance for them. During the process, most organs were removed from the body via an incision in the left side and placed into canopic jars. The flesh was washed with water from the Nile and covered in salt for forty days, and dehydrating materials such as linen and sawdust were used to give shape and mop up moisture. Specific oils were added to the proceedings for their meaning and their properties.* The exact process was never replicated until 2011 when Channel 4 made the documentary *Mummifying Alan*. In this programme, body donor Alan Billis had consented to be the recipient of this procedure after his death, and the team involved a forensic pathologist I've worked with closely many times, Professor Peter Vanezis.

---

* Frankincense and myrrh were involved, and it's said that the fact they were given to the baby Jesus by the Wise Men was a portent of his early death.

But mummification can happen naturally in environments that are very warm and dry. I encountered several naturally mummified cases, frequently from homes which had the heating left on and no access for flies to the cadaver. In the past, one of the most common scenarios was the mummification of babies who, perhaps after being stillborn, were hidden inside the walls of houses by terrified young mothers. We have one such example in the collection at the Pathology Museum, and similar babies are sadly discovered in the fireplaces of old houses quite frequently. Mummification can also happen in cold, dry climates which is why we sometimes find bog bodies – deceased people who've been naturally preserved in peat bogs or similar – thousands of years later, preserved down to their eyelashes.

As a student of decomposition and decay I am familiar with all these stages, yet somewhere a decision seems to have been made about which of these states are suitable for general viewing. When you think about it, the last stage – dry remains – is a much more common sight than bloat or advanced decay. We may see dry remains in museums, on TV documentaries and even in newspaper articles about the latest archaeological find, but we never see maggot-infested corpses strewn around with the same abandon. In fact, the only time this happens is during horror movies, when they are used as a device to scare the bejesus out of us in one way or another. But why is one stage more acceptable for general consumption than the other? Is it because, as Christine Quigley says, 'the skeleton denuded of its facial features has less impact than the preserved head of a mummy, which in turn has less impact than the face of an intact corpse'?

The images of the decomposing deceased, whether via museums or media, are one-dimensional without the accompanying smells, most of which I described above. When discussing the cloying scent of decay the jury is out as to whether it really does cling to your hair and clothes as is so often mentioned in crime books and on TV. I was told by one pathologist that it's not the case. In fact, the delicate odour molecules simply cling to the hairs and folds inside your nasal passages making it seem as though you're smelling it on you all day, but it's from the inside, not the outside.

Perhaps that is true, but often as an APT, once I'd done autopsies and even showered and changed my scrubs, I'd head home in my own clothes and still get a pretty wide berth on the bus.

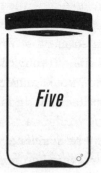

Five

Penetration: 'Rose Cottage'

I know the secrets of love ... It is I who set the
Rose in motion and move the hearts of lovers.
—Farid ud-Din Attar, The Conference of the Birds

Watching someone carry out an autopsy is, in many ways, like watching someone have sex. This is what struck me the very first time I saw one. Before you close this book in misplaced disgust – or, conversely, read on with expectant carnal glee – let me explain.

An autopsy presents as an intimate process between two people: eviscerator and 'evisceratee'. The eviscerator, or technician, removes the organs, the other – the cadaver – is eviscerated. Under normal circumstances a person wouldn't be privy to this activity so it feels forbidden, taboo and voyeuristic. There is a transgressive element to just standing there, watching. There is nudity (the cadaver; hopefully not the technician), body fluids, musky odours and maybe some awkwardness and tentativeness at first. Then hands begin to move deftly across naked flesh, knowing the best moves to make; knowing the dance because it's a dance that's been done a thousand times before. It's an intimacy you feel privileged to be a part of.

The eviscerator may be someone you've seen in person frequently, but never like this. You may have discussed post-mortem procedures over and over again with him during your training, as one discusses sex over and over again with friends, but you've never actually seen him do it. Not until now – the first time – when you're invited to lose your PM room 'virginity' and witness the act in all its technicolour glory. I think the poet-undertaker Thomas Lynch put it best when he said, 'Both sex and death are horizontal mysteries that possess similarly disconcerting effects.' Horizontal, yes. Mysterious, certainly. Disconcerting? Absolutely – for most. But for us in the business of death, the autopsy is a mystery that needs to be solved.

I'd lost my autopsy virginity when I was in university, but everything I'd done in my life had been building up to that moment. During my gap year, serendipity struck for me. My estranged father moved to a large house in Worthing with a self-contained flat in its annexe, and it just so happened a friend's mother, Sarah, was an embalmer at a funeral home in a town not far from Worthing. At around seven months pregnant with a little girl, Sarah needed someone to help her manoeuvre the heavier cadavers and undress them, rather than constantly ask funeral directors at their company, J. Ellwoods and Sons, to assist – they were usually busy with their own tasks. This was the ideal experience for me. Young, strong and very enthusiastic, I slipped into the voluntary role in order to learn all I could about embalming.

While some of my friends took their year out in exotic places, to me it seemed worth heading to an unfamiliar little town on the south coast for a while in order to strengthen family ties as well as gain some experience with the dead and find out if I actually had the stomach for this type of work. So that's what I did. I remember having coffee with my three closest friends a day or two before I hopped on to the train with just one large case and a handbag. We were all the same age and embarking on completely different journeys: one was pregnant, one was heading to live in France and then Spain to study languages, and one was going travelling in South East Asia.

I was off to wash and dress the dead.

This might have been my year off from education, but it was really the period when I learned the most. It was there that I experienced a funeral home for the first time, because I'd been far too young to visit either of my grandparents when they passed away. It was all new to me: the solemn, quiet hallways of J. Ellwoods and Sons, the ever-present soothing scent of flowers, the warmth from the heaters, and the ambient lighting casting shadows that softened every sharp edge. Even people's grief seemed softer here, the general hush instilling a cloistered calm into everyone who passed through. All of this was juxtaposed with the sound of the boisterous boys in the 'back' as they washed down hearses and trimmed coffins, and the tinny radio in Sarah's prep room that belted out popular music that hadn't really been popular since the seventies and eighties. In an unusual way, this was heaven for me, and I never felt uncomfortable. For the first time in my life I was independent, following my dreams, and doing something I'd wanted to do for years. Unlike much of the population, I associate funeral homes with peace and tranquillity. I'd wake up at the crack of dawn to be at J. Ellwoods and Sons a couple of towns away at an early hour, so sometimes, when fatigue hit, I would wander off into one of the suites adjoining the chapels of rest and take a nap on the sofa – obviously only when it wasn't otherwise occupied – much to the distress of the company's long-suffering cleaner who'd often jump out of her skin at my unexpected presence. Spending a drowsy hour on the sofa after helping to prep the decedents gave me time to reflect on what I'd learned and consider my future path. I was at peace there.

Even then I knew that positions in mortuaries opened up very rarely and embalming could be an alternative career for me, or even a skill I could perfect and have under my belt before a job opportunity in a mortuary came about. I learned exactly what an embalmer does, and it's a procedure I passionately believe everyone should know about for two reasons: so that it doesn't get confused with the role of the APT, and so that an informed decision can be made about whether or not you'd like it for a family member, or even yourself, because it's not required by law. Embalming is an aesthetic, cosmetic process that is carried out at the undertaker's, rather than at the mortuary, although it can happen at the family home. Autopsies, on the other hand, can only happen at mortuaries, or specially designated temporary mortuaries in the case of mass fatalities, for example. There's no such thing as a 'home autopsy' or a 'DIY post-mortem' . . . at least, not a legal one.

I didn't know what to expect and I had no idea what spending time with an embalmer, particularly a female one, would be like. One thing missing from B-movie horrors are females in antagonist roles, so I'd always imagined embalmers to be like the weird male scientists seen in those films: Bela Lugosi in *The Corpse Vanishes* or Vincent Price in *Scream and Scream Again* (of course, Sarah was nothing like that). Instead, the only image I associated with Sarah was that of Fenella Fielding in *Carry on Screaming*. It may sound silly but if you've seen the film, in which Fenella's character, Valeria, and her brother carry out a strange procedure on beautiful young living women to turn them into shop mannequins, you might not be entirely surprised to learn that there is actually a similarity when it comes to embalming.

Modern embalming is the process of replacing the deceased's body fluids with preservative chemicals in order to retard decay. It's the story of Pygmalion's statue in reverse; that which was once human and vulnerable becomes serene and azoic – just like in *Carry on Screaming*. It's done so that the vibrant palette and infernal stench of decomposition (see last chapter) isn't witnessed or experienced by the family and friends of the deceased if the funeral requires an open-coffin viewing and the disposal isn't happening for a few days. It's not as common in the UK as it is in the US. But for those who do require it, it will cost extra and is often called 'hygienic treatment', although the term is a bit of a misnomer as the deceased are no more dangerous if they are not embalmed – except in the case of some infectious diseases – which is why it's important to note that it's not required by law. Some funeral directors are very upfront about their costs: they explain that the procedure will add around £150 to the bill

(outside London it can be as low as £70) and they won't perform it unless they receive prior informed consent. Others,
however, will call the procedure 'cosmetic treatment' and rail-
road the bereaved into paying for it at best, or at worst just go
ahead and do it without permission, adding the cost on later.

On my first day at J. Ellwoods and Sons, after I'd satisfied
myself that Sarah was nothing like Valeria from that cheesy
film, I asked her why she'd wanted to be an embalmer. She
simply said 'to help people'. She assured me that at J. Ellwoods
and Sons the procedure was only carried out when families
were fully aware of the costs and requested it themselves.

I wanted to gain some experience myself so I dived straight
in. The case in question was an old lady, around seventy-five,
and nothing too dramatic for a first-timer like me. In the prep
room, heavily pregnant Sarah waddled towards me with the
garments I was soon to become so familiar with: a surgical
cotton gown and plastic apron. While I covered my clothes
she pulled her long, dark Jane Russell hair up over her ample
bosom and into a ponytail, then swaddled her swollen belly
with a green plastic apron stretched so taut around the bump
that horizontal white streaks appeared. She seemed glamorous and competent, and younger than her forty-odd years,
but maybe it was the pregnancy glow giving her a youthful
aura? It struck me as odd to have so many archetypal stages
of female development in one room: the unborn baby, myself
as The Maiden, Sarah as The Mother and the deceased as The
Crone,* all of us overshadowed by the final, unapologetic
figure of Death itself.

---

* Maiden, Mother and Crone are pagan archetypes used to describe the stages in a
woman's life as well as the three faces of the moon: waxing, full and waning.

Sarah told me to pop some gloves on and instructed me to just feel the hand of the deceased. 'It's important to get used to the cold,' she said. 'It can be a bit strange initially.' I reached out tentatively to touch, for the first time, someone who had died, acutely aware that I was crossing a boundary. Not only was I about to have an experience there was no going back from, I also realised I was doing so without the consent of the woman on Sarah's table. Yes, I was only touching her hand, but she wasn't present to tell me whether or not I had permission to, so I had to project it to her myself, mentally explaining that I was part of the embalming procedure – the process her family had agreed to – and it was therefore not a violation. And while her cold hand was in mine I realised I had never held my own nan's hand. Never. I couldn't, not with those weird brown arthritis contraptions she used to wear on both wrists, her twisted fingers popping out of the tops like curled twigs. Instead, I had this moment of intimacy with a stranger.

The lady had been in the fridge for a while and the skin of her hand was firm like pale putty, yet cooler than a pint of milk. Sarah was right – I'd never felt anything quite like it. I had the sense of dipping my toe into very cold water, and even after I'd removed it the cold remained – a constant reminder of that other subterranean world.

It was time to undress the deceased, which is usually the first part of the embalming process, as the existing clothes may be soiled. Families tend to bring in new clothes for their loved ones to be buried or cremated in: their best outfit or something they may even have picked out themselves. It seems like a simple and practical step but, as Christine Quigley puts it, 'the withered body of a cadaver, minus clothing and eyeglasses, provokes the distancing necessary to cut it up'. With the accoutrements of life removed, the task is easier both practically and psychologically.

So this would be my first time undressing someone who was dead, and again there was that sense of transgressive intimacy: I had seen few people naked in my life, yet here I was with a naked stranger.

Soon we began the embalming, which is nothing like the Ancient Egyptians' process and doesn't even have the same principles. Sarah gestured to a huge vat of cheerful pastel-coloured liquid. 'All the blood in their veins and fluid in their cells needs to be replaced with this,' she said. The fluid, a concoction of formaldehyde, methanol and other solvents, is mixed in a pump and is usually a pink- or peach-coloured milkshake with a name like 'natural tone' or 'perfect tone'. It reminded me of vintage pancake make-up; sickly sweet. Sarah bent down and deftly made an incision into the neck with a scalpel, causing me to take an involuntary step back, assuming I was going to be sprayed with blood. Of course, there was no blood flow, as the heart had stopped long ago, so I was able to inch forward and bend over to take a closer look. What I saw was just like in my anatomy books. Well, the vein wasn't blue and the artery red like in many of those typical medical illustrations, but to me the different layers of the flesh were distinct enough: the muscle, the fat and the vessels Sarah was incising with the scalpel. She easily made another incision directly into the carotid artery and inserted a thin metal pipe linked to a rubber tube and the huge vat of pinky-peach liquid. A different tube and pipe were inserted into the jugular vein for drainage. Once the pump was turned on, the pastel fluid was forced into the arteries, at the same time pushing the blood out, or displacing it. This process not only removes bacteria in the vessels and therefore most of the cells of the body as it seeps into them via the capillaries, it also gives the flesh a more lifelike tone; there are slightly different colours of fluids for the vast ranges of different skin tones. It even changes how the skin feels, creating plumpness and curves which will eventually harden or 'set'. I had to massage the limbs as the fluid flowed to ensure an even distribution, again creating an intimacy I hadn't anticipated.

Once that was complete and the last of the woman's bodily fluids had gurgled down the drain, I thought that was the end of the fluid part. But then Sarah pulled out what looked like a long metal sword attached to a rubber tube, and I guessed it was the trocar. This is an aspirating tool which I'd read about during my research. It had a sharp pointed end with lots of tiny holes around it and the idea was to perforate the abdomen and the organs, then suck fluids through the holes and into the pump. But the words 'perforate' and 'aspirate' sound more clinical than the procedure actually looks. Sarah appeared to be practising her fencing technique as she repeatedly inserted the sharp point through the skin of the abdomen and manoeuvred it at different angles, jabbing through the maze of organs. Simultaneously, fluids and gases were pulled up through the trocar and into the collecting drum with a hissing, gurgling sound, just like someone draining the dregs of a drink from a paper cup with a straw. Then the reverse occurred as preservative was introduced into the abdominal cavity in place of the fluids, creating a sort of viscera chutney.

The trocar has become synonymous with the embalmer. The word comes from the French *trois-quarts*, which means 'three quarts'. It was historically used on the living to relieve the pressure caused by a build-up of fluids – oedema – or gases in the belly, so the 'three quarts' likely refers to the amount of substance removed during its use. A 'quart' is two pints so that's a heck of a lot of fluid, or gas, and should give you an idea how much I swallowed during my ill-fated first bloated decomp.

The holes in the abdomen left by the trocar insertion are either stitched up or tiny plastic trocar buttons are popped in to ensure there is no fluid leakage, and with all these buttons and thick stitches I felt like I was in a craft class. In a similar attempt to prevent leakage, Sarah also introduced cotton wool to the nostrils of the patient with forceps ('to stop any purge', she explained) then asked me to gently turn the deceased on her side so she could add some to the rectum for the same purpose. It was an odd sight, this young woman thrusting reams and reams of white cotton wool into the old lady's anus while chatting about everyday things.

'How are you finding living in Worthing so far?' she asked me as a huge wad of white fluff and the end of the long forceps disappeared about a hand's length into the woman's anal cavity.

'Great.' I couldn't say much more than that, I was a bit mesmerised.

'Nice to be by the sea air, isn't it?' *Thrust.* 'I'm from Liverpool too and I feel the difference. It's just so much fresher down here.' *Thrust.*

'Hmmmm,' I managed to agree.

When the thrusting was over, of course it crossed my mind

it was a bit undignified. But then I'd had cotton wool shoved into my mouth at the dentist's, and suffered worse indignities at the hands of a gynaecologist, so perhaps that's just what it means to be a human? Even in death we remain a patient: we leak and we excrete. We can't just ignore that and hope for the best.

Finally, we dressed the old lady in fresh clothes (which remained fresh, thanks to all that cotton wool) and Sarah used special non-thermogenic make-up to create the illusion of life. This make-up, unlike our thermogenic make-up, is not made to react with heat from the face. When finished, the decedent looked as though she was sleeping. The process only took about two hours, a lot less time than the Egyptians allocated to their process, and the embalmed woman had been treated as though she was on her way to some big celebration, not her own funeral. Many times after that experience, when I was beautifying myself for a date – applying make-up and choosing just the right outfit – it occurred to me I may well go to the same trouble for my funeral one day.

The current embalming method, and the one I assisted Sarah with all those years ago, involves a series of stages which may appear a bit unseemly. But the upside is that some decedents can be made to look much more at peace and presentable, certainly in cases of disfigurement or advancing decomposition, which theoretically smoothes the path for the next of kin's grief. It's a double-edged sword – or trocar.

If the deceased has a slightly damaged or dainty circulatory system the incision process may be repeated on other parts of the body, for example, the femoral artery in the leg or axillary in the armpit. In the case of an autopsied body, the procedure is more difficult as the circulatory system has been compromised by organ removal. In that instance a six-point injection will be used, meaning embalming fluid is introduced via arteries in both sides of the neck, both armpits and both legs. The viscera bag containing the organs simply has fluid poured into it and is placed back into the cavity before the deceased is stitched up and the rest of the procedure completed as usual. Once the person is in the coffin the embalmer has, in some ways, worked a little bit of magic.

In the twenty-first century the Western world seems to be taking this obsession with looking good after death too far. Embalming, which began during the American Civil War as a way for dead soldiers to be preserved long enough to allow them to return home for burial, has become a cosmetic and almost miraculous procedure. Families aren't usually told the process will only delay decomposition; they're given the impression it will stop it completely, leaving the deceased intact in their grave like an incorruptible holy relic. The process, with the embalmer being given the deceased's own make-up (to compare shades) or hair products and photos of them in life to create as much realism as possible, has advanced. According to historian Brandy Schillace, the Victorians went to great lengths to ensure the deceased looked better in death than in life, even using false teeth and fake, dyed hair. More recently, there is a bizarre form of cosmetic surgery whereby customers are asking for prepaid funeral plans that include filler injections in their lips and collagen in their wrinkles to ensure they look good on their big day. If you can't afford this type of treatment you could pay for famous make-up brand Illamasqua to do your post-mortem make-up rather than the embalmer – at a cost of £450! But just who are these good-looking corpses trying to impress?

In Austria, the cult of the good-looking dead is known as *Schöne Leiche*, or the 'Beautiful Corpse'. Its goal is an aesthetically pleasing focus of the funeral – the deceased – as well as a grand, luxurious send-off with lots of mourners, insinuating that good looks, wealth, popularity and a lasting memorial all go hand in hand. It's certainly not a new concept – after all, Egyptian pyramids and ancient embalming techniques are evidence of the human desire to make a good impression, even when dead. In fact, the word 'mausoleum' comes to us via King Mausolus of Asia Minor for whom, after his death, a huge and extravagant tomb was created in Halicarnassus (now Bodrum), Turkey. The word 'mausoleum' then became synonymous with any grand resting place. It seems that, as well as leaving a legacy of grandeur, everyone wants to walk through those pearly gates looking their very best. One of the more famous advocates of perfect post-mortem make-up was Marilyn Monroe. Her beauty routine, while alive, took up to three hours and she only ever had one make-up artist from her first screen test in 1946 right to the end of her life, Allan 'Whitey' Snyder. They developed such a close relationship she asked him to do her funeral make-up in the event she died before him, a promise he fulfilled in 1962.

I never needed to go and train as an embalmer as I acquired my dream job straight out of university. Becoming a trainee APT was my first full-time job, and as I settled into the routine and began receiving a steady wage, I embraced my independence once more and decided it was time to move out of the family home. A lovely little flat became available on a street within walking distance of where I'd been brought up and it was immediately opposite my gym: it was *perfect*. The road was Rose Lane, and the flat, instead of having a number, was called 'Rose Cottage'. When I told June at work one day she couldn't believe it.

'Yer what?' she exclaimed. 'Rose Cottage?'

'Yeah ... what's wrong with that?' I countered, taken aback by her tone.

June would sometimes take off her glasses and wipe them on her scrubs when she wanted to drag a moment out. She had a lot to teach me so there were a lot of moments to drag out. Like this one.

'Rose Cottage means "mortuary" in hospitals, ya know, Tiny,' she said with a knowing look. She put her glasses back on. 'And here's you moving into one!'

I hadn't known that, having not yet worked in a hospital mortuary at that point in my career. What a coincidence, though: Rose Cottage, the first home for the fledgling mortician.

I've since thought about the association with roses a little more, and I still find it unusual that these particular flowers are used in this euphemism, given how they represent love and sex. Roses are often symbolic of female genitalia, and the Ancient Greeks and Romans associated them with their goddesses of love, Aphrodite and Venus respectively. But the rose is also said to have bloomed from the blood of the crucified Christ, when heavy drops fell on to the parched ground, symbolising death and sacrifice. Its beautiful petals, which may be the colour of blood or flesh, can hide dangerous thorns which are perfectly placed to draw blood. The rose also speaks of secrets: in Ancient Rome one would be placed at the site of a confidential meeting or activity. To that effect, *sub rosa*, or 'beneath the rose', means something clandestine – 'keep it quiet'. Perhaps this is what the rose of Rose Cottage speaks of? After all, mortuaries are normally hidden from view in hospitals and not clearly signposted. There are two fears: that a normal person will come to the mortuary and be traumatised, or that a weirdo will come to the mortuary for some lascivious reason. There seems to be no happy medium.

The Municipal Mortuary I worked in had its hidden entrance down an alleyway because it was tucked in behind one of the buildings of the medical school. This meant it was ideally placed for me to go and receive my first inoculations in years for hepatitis, tuberculosis and meningitis – a precaution against infection, along with all that PPE. But it also meant that it was used by people to carry out rather nefarious activities, normally once we'd gone home. Many were the mornings we'd find used condoms on our front step, those two bedfellows, sex and death, having united under the cover of darkness (probably prostitutes 'carrying out transactions' with their customers, although it may well have been couples enjoying each other after a night in one of the nearby bars). But all of the used condoms were a far better sight than the one time I arrived to discover a perfect spiral of human faeces on the stoop. Was it deliberate, perhaps someone expressing distaste for what went on in this tiny building hidden away

from the road? Probably not, but evidently our *sub rosa* location wasn't necessarily a positive thing.

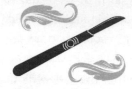

Back in the PM room in our *sub rosa* building, once the tools
had been prepared and the external examination had been
carried out, I would take up a shiny new PM40. I'd bend over
the deceased and make the first cut just like I had all that
time ago under Jason's supervision. I'd penetrate the flesh
of the neck and slide the blade all the way down to the pubic
bone to create the Y-incision. The cuts would open slightly
like thin yellow smiles, since mainly golden adipose tissue
is visible between the layers of skin. Often, and particularly
if my case was someone frail because they were either young
or very old, I'd place my gloved left hand on the forehead to
steady them as I made the incision with my right. Sometimes
it seemed perhaps too tender a gesture, out of place in such an
environment, but it was a way to comfort someone who was
about to undergo a procedure that many still consider a violation, and perhaps minimise the indignities of the patient at
this final port of call. The person to be autopsied is dead and
what remains may be just a shell, but that never stops us, the
people who work with the deceased, considering them something 'other'. When dealing with the dead I was constantly
reminded of Thomas Lynch's words: 'The bodies of the newly
dead are not debris nor remnant, nor are they entirely icon or
essence. They are, rather, changelings, incubates, hatchlings

of a new reality ... It is wise to treat such new things tenderly, carefully, with honour.'

And just what if, at that particular point of penetration, the deceased woke up? Would that touch give them comfort? Perhaps their eyes fly open, they scream, or they reflexively reach out and clasp the scalpel-wielder's wrist in a cadaveric death grip. I know that this is highly improbable but anecdotally it does happen – tales abound of people waking up in the mortuary, 'on the slab', even in coffins. As recently as November 2014, a ninety-one-year-old Polish woman, Janina Kolkiewicz, woke up in a mortuary eleven hours after being declared dead. In January 2014, Paul Mutora woke up in a morgue in Kenya, fifteen hours after swallowing insecticide, and in March of the same year, Walter Williams came to in a body bag at a funeral home in Mississippi. Perhaps most unbelievable was the Russian man who woke up in a morgue in December 2015 after drinking copious amounts of vodka, only to go back to the party and continue drinking! Spoiler alert: those people were never actually dead.

I once worked with a doctor who joked that with the first plunge of his blade into the neck of one of his cases he knew she'd been alive because of the unexpected spurt of her carotid blood. As I found out during my first embalming, the recently deceased do have most of their blood, but it doesn't shoot out like it would in a live patient. Firstly, there's no working pump – the heart – to force it around the body, and secondly, the blood begins to solidify or coagulate from the moment of death, settling into that reddish-purple hypostasis. When this doctor was asked by his technician at the time 'Good God, was she even dead?', he'd apparently quipped, 'Well, she is *now*.'

It's an implausible story – although perhaps it makes a good tale for him to tell at dinner parties – yet it's not the only one I've heard, and not the most disturbing. An APT in a mortuary in northern England told me of a pathologist he knew, a borderline sadistic man who used to take pleasure in thrusting a thermometer into the vaginas of deceased females 'to take their internal temperature' (I put that in quotation marks because the correct way to do that is with an incision into the liver). On one occasion his female decedent, who had been removed from a freezing river, was given the typical thermometer treatment, only this time an onlooker noticed a thin, silver tear slide out of her open eye and down onto the steel tray. The insinuation was that she hadn't been dead, and instead was in a hypothermic state from her body shutting down in the river, yet evidently able to cry at the painful violation.

These are just stories I have heard over the years I've been working in the industry, urban legends; I have no way of knowing if there is even a kernel of truth in them. But the issue isn't about people being resurrected and brought back to life so much as people being mistaken for being dead in the first place. In the book *How We Die*, Sherwin B. Nuland says that the 'appearance of a newly lifeless face cannot be mistaken for unconsciousness', but this is evidently not the case. The effect of extreme cold on the body can place it in a sort of suspended animation and it can be difficult to tell if the victim truly is deceased. Many examples of this preservation and recovery exist, from those drowning in icy water to others becoming suffocated beneath an avalanche, or simply falling unconscious and hypothermic until they are found and (hopefully) revived. But how they are revived can also be an issue. You wouldn't want to be brought back to consciousness via the sting of a pathologist's scalpel cutting through your carotid.

Perhaps the most disturbing case was in Romania in 1992, when an eighteen-year-old 'dead' female was brought back to life as she was being raped by a necrophilic mortuary worker. He was arrested, but the parents were so grateful to him for 'resurrecting' their daughter they refused to press charges, saying she 'owed him her life'. Sex and death entwined once again.

Suffice to say I've never experienced any of *my* patients waking up, but there are certainly tricks to this effect that seasoned technicians and mortuary managers used to play on their newbies. For example, I heard tales of one ringleader constantly playing the same joke on their trainees. He'd get into a body bag in the cold store and have his right-hand man close him into the fridge. Then, when the trainee was being given the tour, the fridge door would be opened and the 'body' pulled out only for it to sit up and scream, scaring the impressionable newbie half to death. My favourite part of this story is when, one year, one of the more junior APTs decided to get revenge. The trick was carried out as usual, but unbeknown to the ringleader hiding in his body bag, the bag next to him in the fridge was also occupied ... by the vengeful junior. As Mr Joker lay in the fridge, probably suppressing a laugh, ready to be pulled out to perform for the umpteenth time, the bag next to him started writhing and groaning in the darkness. He jumped so high he cracked his forehead open on the tray above him and never attempted that prank again.

One of my favourite quotes comes from Caleb Wilde, a sixth-generation undertaker from the US who blogs about his experiences. 'As a mortician,' he said, 'I always tie the shoe-laces together of the dead. Because if there is ever a zombie apocalypse, it will be hilarious.' This is what we in the trade call 'gallows humour'.

Thankfully, I've never experienced knocking from the inside of the cold store, hands grabbing my PM40, or any shuffling dead. But most of all the deceased do still remain human and in some cases seem 'alive'. Positioned precariously on top of head blocks, they may slowly turn towards you. As I mentioned, they may groan, burp or fart. Sometimes tiny air bubbles of blood pop out of the nose, giving the appearance of breathing, just like the cat had done all those years ago. As Mary Roach mentioned in her bestseller *Stiff*, 'cadavers occasionally affect a sort of accidental humanness which catches the medical professional off guard'. She describes an anatomy student who had the unnerving experience of a corpse's arm around her waist. I discovered this myself frequently: when I'd lift an arm in full rigor over the deceased's head and turn my back to wash down the side of the body, slowly, without me seeing it, the arm would circle back round again until suddenly I'd feel a cold hand on the warm flesh of my bottom, through my scrubs.

Back in the post-mortem room, once the incision had been made and the deceased had stayed (thankfully) lifeless and quiet through the whole ordeal, the next stage was to separate the skin of the chest from the ribs. This was always described by the people who trained me as 'like filleting a fish', which was most unhelpful as I'd never filleted a fish. I'd just nod my head and watch intently until eventually I had the knack.

Holding the skin flap in one hand I'd very gently pull it at the same time as touching the knife to the strands of white connective tissue being stretched taut by the action. This strips the skin away from the bone of the ribs and the intercostal muscle until it falls to the side like an open pyjama top on someone lying in bed. After repeating the action on the other side I'd be left with a wide V-shaped window through which I could see the striations of white and red as the ribs and intercostal muscles descended from the neck down, like steps on a ladder.

They abruptly come to a stop halfway down, giving way to a large, flat mass of bobbly yellow substance called the omentum. This is a sort of 'fat flap' which hangs down over the abdominal organs like a golden apron, protecting them. It's attached at the top to the large intestine which sweeps from left to right, beneath the diaphragm, but it's not attached at the bottom, it just lays over all the intestines then tucks down into the pelvis, keeping everything neat and safe.

This neatness, this perfect biological jigsaw, reminded me of the anatomical models I'd become familiar with during my years of study: those plastic, headless torsos I'd encountered at museums and at school, with organs that would pop out easily to reveal a shiny smooth cavity with little metal hooks inside to keep the pieces in place. But long before those armless, decapitated figures became the staple of every anatomical classroom or film set, some students used the Anatomical Venus to learn their subject.

These Venuses, made from wax and looking incredibly lifelike, were popular in the eighteenth century because they were a means for students to study anatomy despite the shortage of cadavers, and without having to get involved with the associated ethical restrictions of employing body snatchers. There was also no odour or icky fluid to deal with, something which the prospective doctors no doubt welcomed. But the unusual thing about these particular anatomical models is they were more often than not deliberately created in the form of a beautiful woman – they actually had arms and a head for a start. Some gorgeous examples are still on display and I'm lucky enough to have seen them in real life in both La Specola in Florence and the Josephinum in Vienna. They recline lasciviously in glass cases, often on velvet or satin cushions, and from the top of the head down they look like pretty shop mannequins, although instead of wearing clothes they wear a look of post-orgasmic bliss. This odalisque-like appearance is enhanced by their long flowing real hair, realistic glass eyes (half-open, which suggests life as opposed to death) and even pearl necklaces, tiaras or other jewellery.* This abruptly changes at the level of the sternum, however, when the torso blooms into an open cavity of organs like petals in dark red, dark yellow and brown. These organs, also made from wax, could be removed one by one and handled by the onlooker in the same manner as our current plastic models. Usually, once the uterus was exposed and opened it would even reveal an angelic foetus curled up inside.

These Anatomical Venuses, also called 'Slashed Beauties' and 'Dissected Graces', were objects at the interface of art and science. They were ostensibly used to demonstrate anatomy to a male student body, which may have had some bearing on their pleasing appearance. Perhaps it was less traumatic for the students to be faced with their own death

---

* Incidentally, they have pubic hair – *real* pubic hair, shaved from cadavers and added to the model – yet no underarm hair. I suppose they have their own 'waxers'? Bah-bum-chhhhh.

in the form of a figure of the opposite sex? They certainly would identify with it less, unlike when I encountered the female prosthetic on the film set and saw myself in her unkempt hair and smooth skin. Perhaps it was simply an attempt to buffer an unpleasant image with an attractive casing? But these Venuses were also used to illustrate God's ability to create, not only the beauty on the outside but also the intricacies of the organs within. Whatever the reason for these perfect models, the audience is certainly confronted, in one arresting glance, by all the mysteries of life, sex and death.

But why are sex and death considered bedfellows? Most logically, the connection is that sex begins life and death ends it – a circle of life. The French call an orgasm *la petite mort*, or 'the little death', perhaps in honour of this association between the two great mysteries of life. Some creatures actually enter into a frenzy of mating that begins in sex and ends in death, and stories of fictional teens falling in love with the 'undead' saturate modern media.

Often we have to lighten the mood in the PM room with a joke or two, no matter how serious a doctor might be, and it can be gallows humour, or perhaps a bit more *Carry On Mortuary*. One day, while assisting on the autopsy of a man with heart failure, I noticed that one of the fingers on his left hand was white compared to the other more pink ones.

'What on earth is *that*?' I asked Dr Jameson, who was half-way through the external exam.

He took a quick look. 'Oh, that's Vibration White Finger,' he said, nonchalantly.

'Vibration White Finger?'

I couldn't wrap my head around it, so he elaborated: 'It's a blood flow issue, a type of Raynaud's disease caused by pro-longed use of vibrating equipment.'

My head shot up in alarm and he suddenly burst out laughing. 'No, not *those* types of vibrating tools,' he remarked, with a wink.

I went utterly crimson.

To make it worse, he added, 'Are you using hydraulic drills in bed?'

I shook my head, trying not to catch his eye.

'Then you'll be fine,' he chuckled, and cracked on with the dissection as though nothing had happened.

I, meanwhile, wanted the mortuary floor to swallow me whole.

I discovered early on as an APT that the connection between sex and death is not only symbolic but also literal, when I encountered my first auto-erotic asphyxiation case.

'Whatever you see here, you can't tell anybody about it,' Andrew said to me one day, with a solemn expression on his face.

Andrew's face was far too expressive. Every thought he had slid across his features like a dark cloud across the sky, and it was often disconcerting to have a conversation with him. He was so pleasant when he was in a good mood and his features relaxed into a smile, but it just didn't happen often. This particular grim expression lent a note of seriousness to the morning's proceedings.

Opening the body bag with trepidation I was faced with a sight I'd sadly already become familiar with: a man, face bloated, tongue protruding, a noose tied tight around his neck. But this one was slightly different to the hanging cases

I'd seen before. There were some socks between the noose and the skin of his neck.

'What are the socks for?' I asked Andrew, my eyebrows raised in surprise. (Perhaps his animated facial expressions were contagious?)

'Auto-erotic asphyxiation,' he explained. 'Because he wasn't actually trying to kill himself he used the socks to take some of the pressure off the noose and avoid visible rope burns.'

Makes sense, I thought, but I didn't ask Andrew why he knew so much about it . . .

Once the body bag was removed, it became clear this wasn't an attempted suicide but a sex-game gone wrong. the deceased was wearing women's knickers and stockings. I did wonder if perhaps he had been murdered and set up – I mean, what an utterly embarrassing way to go. If you wanted to really dig the knife in after murdering your enemy you might truss them up to make sure they looked like they'd been doing something like this. But the pathologist reassured me it was unlikely. For a start, there are ways to tell when a person has hanged himself, often to do with the angle left by the noose around the neck. Then there's the circumstantial evidence: drug use, hotel room booked under a pseudonym, porn on the TV, etc.

'All very typical, very common features,' said the pathologist.

'Common?' I exclaimed. 'How common *is* it?'

I discovered it's a difficult question to answer. Although, as I've said, the Coroner in the UK does not perform post-mortems, he is an important part of the procedure as he oversees the inquests. These public, legal inquiries are some-times opened in the case of unnatural deaths so that the

Coroner can establish the cause. He simply has to answer four questions: who was the deceased, and how, when and where did they die? In a suspected case of auto-erotic asphyxiation the question of 'how' can cause problems. The family may be upset at a verdict of 'misadventure' as it implies something unusual, and the Coroner may not be 100 per cent sure the death was intended so he may not want to label it suicide. Therefore, the verdict is often left as 'open'. This means that gleaning statistics of these types of death can be difficult. That said, it has been estimated that five hundred to a thousand men die every year in the US from this practice, but far fewer women. UK figures are harder to come by.

In these cases, it is the external exam that gives most of the information, the attire and the neck wound being most important. Then, of course, circumstances of death add pieces to the puzzle. So why have an autopsy at all? If it's so obvious from the outside, can't we just say on the certificate 'death by hanging' and leave it at that? We can't for two reasons. Firstly, there may well be an underlying health condition in the patient. Perhaps the person who diced with death and practised auto-erotic asphyxiation had a reason to throw caution to the wind; maybe he had a terminal illness he'd told nobody about, or perhaps didn't know about himself. HIV for example, or a form of cancer? This may be useful for next of kin or previous partners to know. Secondly, the World Health Organisation also needs to know these statistics so that they're informed of the major health conditions people are commonly suffering from, and therefore where to invest money for treatment. An autopsy is not just to establish immediate cause of death, it contributes to a body of knowledge used by the whole world.

And then, of course, there's the odd surprise. When we opened up the case that morning we found a butt plug that had entered the man's rectum so far we hadn't noticed it during the external examination. I removed it as it seemed more dignified to bury the man without it in there, and I was used to pulling things out by now after thrusting so much cotton wool into patients like I'd seen Sarah do years earlier. But I really didn't want to be the one to hand it over to the family with the man's personal effects. How would they feel? Ultimately, our aim is to allow the deceased to leave the premises in the best shape possible and as close to their natural state as possible, interfering as little as we can with the perfection of the outside and inside of the deceased. A butt plug doesn't come into the equation of 'natural state', but after I placed it in a sealed plastic bag I did stand in the mortuary, holding it by the corner, for an inordinately long amount of time, while I tried to work out what on earth to do with it.

The stunning thing about the human body is that every tissue looks different yet every single one has a purpose and a place, even the strange flap of yellow omentum providing a safety blanket for the organs. It's a marvel of design and engineering, even if it can be artificially manipulated by ropes around the neck and foreign objects inside orifices.

This, then, is the landscape of the human body at the first frontier. Sometimes after that initial incision – the moment the curtains of the flesh are pulled back to reveal the ribs – there will be evident pathology to help identify cause of death: perhaps lots of yellow fluid called ascites in the abdomen, or perhaps some angry red criss-cross rib fractures. Other times, as Elisabeth Bronfen said, 'Cutting into the body, entering the labyrinth of Otherness, may in fact only lead back to an encounter with oneself . . . ' Either way, you're now inside and there's no turning back. The only option is to go in deeper.

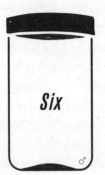

Thoracic Block:
'Home Isn't Where the Heart Is'

I am my heart's undertaker. Daily I go and
retrieve its tattered remains, place them
delicately into its little coffin, and bury it in the
depths of my memory, only to have to do it all
again tomorrow.

—*Emilie Autumn*,
The Asylum for Wayward Victorian Girls

I watch horror movies quite frequently and often the lazy plot twist will be 'This house was built on an Indian burial ground!' or 'This orphanage used to be an asylum!' and of course that explains why the child became possessed or the closet contains an opening to hell, blah blah.

These storylines don't scare me.

When I first moved to London I lived just past the grave-yard, round the corner from the prison and opposite the mental hospital. Throw in an Indian burial ground and my life would have been the ideal Halloween TV special. But, I digress. Just what made me leave my relatively safe and small hometown and try my luck in a horror movie cliché? Partly it was a desire to train more, 'to go in deeper', to be promoted somewhere as a now-qualified APT and not just be paid and treated as a 'mortuary assistant-slash-trainee'. But more than that, it was due to one life-changing event.

The morning of Thursday, 7 July 2005 is so fresh in my mind it may as well be yesterday. June and I were in the PM room around eight a.m. with one case each as Andrew took his usual seat in the office chair at his PC – he was finishing up paperwork before heading off on leave. June and I weren't listening to the radio; we'd started proceedings by arguing about whether we'd play my Arcade Fire CD – again, as I'd recently become obsessed with the band – or whether June would finally win out and instead get to listen to the Hannibal Lecter theme composed originally by Bach. She won this time; it was only fair.

While we were carrying out our external examinations to prepare for the pathologist to arrive a little later, we were interrupted by his premature, flustered entrance. Dr Sam Williams, tall and lanky with an air of typical English 'properness', was always a bit awkward, but on this occasion his flurry of activity caused both me and June to cease our banter and lower our clipboards. He dropped his papers and briefcase, stopped the CD and flipped the hi-fi to the radio.

'Haven't you two heard what's going on?'

'No – what?' June asked, bewildered.

'We've been in here since about seven thirty,' I added. 'We haven't got a clue.'

When you're in the isolated PM room focusing on autopsies, the rest of the world may as well not exist.

'There's been an explosion in London,' he informed us, looking pale. 'It might even be two. They think more than one can't be just an accident.'

We didn't really know what to assume but we knew we had to keep working on the patients at hand who deserved our full attention. Still, we left the radio on in the background to find out exactly what was going on. We all had friends and family in London, we were all worried about the situation, and we wanted to know what was happening. We never normally carried out post-mortems in silence: there was usually constant banter about the cases or what we'd been up to the night before. This time, though, there was no talking from us, only the drone of the small radio in the corner of the room echoing off the bare walls and floor tiles.

As time unfolded, like the skin on the torsos of our deceased patients, the truth was revealed, just like their ribs and organs. There had been a terror attack in Britain's capital which had effectively brought it to a standstill. Due to the fact that four bombs had detonated in separate areas of the city, communication lines were down and no one knew for hours if their friends or relatives were safe. It was a cataclysm the like of which our generation in Britain had never experienced.

By the end of that afternoon I had been recruited to go to London and work in the temporary mortuary which was in the process of being set up as part of 'Operation Theseus'. All four bombing sites were to be investigated and their remains to be brought to one central mortuary facility large enough to accommodate the evidence and the victims, as well as the huge number of staff who would need to be involved in this gargantuan investigation: APTs, pathologists, anthropologists, radiographers, DVI (disaster victim identification) teams, SO13 (the Anti-Terrorist Branch as it was at the time), Interpol and more. It was a purpose-built complex of marquees and temporary buildings set up at a barracks in central London in accordance with previously devised emergency preparedness plans. Construction began by the end of that fateful Thursday and it was expected to be fully functional as early as the following day.

I was recruited because I'd put my name forward to be part of a team for emergency alerts in case such an incident should happen in the UK. There is a similar US organisation to the one I'd joined and it's called D-MORT, the 'Disaster Mortuary Operations Response Team'. Great acronym! It practically explains what it is without you even needing to know all the words; it sounds like it could require its members to wear *X-Men*-style uniforms. And what was ours called in the UK? The 'Forensic Response Team', or FRT. Throw in the word 'anatomical' and I would have been working for FART. I wished it was called something as descriptive and snappy as D-MORT but still, a rose by any other name etc. I've since come to realise that clever puns or abbreviations aren't respected by those who don't understand the power they can have when attempting to engage people with a topic. Suffice to say, by the time I was using the word 'technologist' in the wrong context and working for FART, I was already becoming a bit disillusioned and hoping to progress far enough up the professional chain to be a part of the decision-making process in future.

Regardless, being involved in this mass fatality investigation was something akin to being called into a religious order for me. I had studied mass disasters and graves as part of forensic anthropology courses, been to conferences on Disaster Response and was a member of Amnesty International, attending meetings and keeping up to date with global conflicts. I'd read books on mass excavations in the former Yugoslavia and Rwanda and knew there was a possibility of carrying out such work as an APT. Now, suddenly, it was my turn to do something important. I was so grateful. I didn't want to just helplessly watch events unfold on TV. I felt honoured to be given this opportunity to use my training and do something for those who needed it most.

Andrew had left by the end of the working week bound for warmer climes, which left only myself and acting manager, June, in the mortuary. I was incredibly thankful to her for letting me go. I arrived in London on the morning of Saturday, 9 July, having flown into City Airport from Liverpool at seven a.m. as it was a lot quicker than taking the train. I was at the Honourable Artillery Company barracks by eight, and half of the APTs, mostly the London and southern-based ones, were already there. I'd brought my own kit with me: the all-important face visors I was so used to working with, my white nurse's clogs with my name written on which I'd wear daily in our mortuary, and my own set of scrubs just in case. I also had clothes and toiletries; the usual for a few days away. Although we were all being accommodated in the same hotel, there was no time to take those bags to my room. I was instructed to put them in the corner along with everyone else's and then I went straight into the recently erected changing cubicle to throw on some provided scrubs and start work.

The victims were already being brought in and I was amazed that the system was running like clockwork, with teams of people contributing to one well-oiled machine. Each decedent was first X-rayed inside the body bag, with a pathologist overseeing the process, so that pieces of debris that were either dangerous (for example shrapnel) or pivotal to the investigation (for example parts of the bombs) could be recorded in situ then removed carefully. After bag and detritus removal the deceased was then X-rayed again, still under the pathologist's supervision, with just clothing on, to ensure that nothing important had been missed.

Then the victims were transported to the APTs, with the pathologists joining us, working at four autopsy bays in small teams. The teams consisted of the pathologist, two APTs, a photographer and evidence collector from the police force and a member of SO13 – more members than for a routine autopsy but perhaps similar to a forensic post-mortem. We APTs assisted with the removal of the clothing and jewellery, as photographs were taken and personal effects were collected to be labelled with DVI numbers. Once in a blue moon we struck gold and were able to identify victims using their wallets, but most of the time it was more difficult.

It is perhaps obvious that I can't go into too much detail, as it was a sensitive operation and family members who lost loved ones are still grieving, while victims are still suffering from their injuries. It would be careless and cruel for me to reveal too much about what went on.

The days at the facility were intense. We'd begin at seven a.m. or thereabouts and end around seven or eight p.m., at which point we'd have to clean down the whole mortuary ready for the next day. I'd brought enough luggage and clothing for a few days, yet two weeks later I was still there. The APTs working together so tightly under such circumstances became incredibly close: we were all staying at the same hotel, eating meals together, spending all day together then going home together to 'debrief' – by which I mean a drink in the bar and a discussion of the day's events as an emotional outlet. It was here that I met Danny and Chris, the managers from the Metropolitan Hospital in London. They were vivacious and raucous and so different to Andrew in terms of how they managed their younger APTs, Josh and Ryan. They were constantly playing practical jokes and talking about their hilarious escapades. They were able to keep my spirits up through the process of autopsying larger human fragments until finally we were examining small fragments and the forensic anthropologists took over. Then, it was time for me to go home.

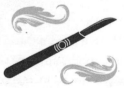

Six difficult months after the terror attacks, once I was back in the Municipal Mortuary and the intensity of the days at the barracks had left me, I was in a dilemma: I wasn't sure if I was happy that things had calmed down or if I was missing the excitement of doing something that felt more worthwhile in a busier place. A position suddenly opened up at the Metropolitan Hospital for a qualified APT with the Certificate. Danny and Chris, remembering me from our time together following 7/7, contacted me to give me the heads-up and see if I wanted to apply.

Had I thought of moving? Had I thought of working in a hospital rather than a Coronial mortuary? Did I want to work towards my Diploma?

Yes to all these questions. Yes, yes, yes. I suppose that answered my dilemma.

I applied, and I got the job.

Even with my eyes closed, I always knew when I'd stepped off the train, through the doors of Euston Station and into London. Compared to the north, the air had an oppressive quality; perhaps because the temperature was always a degree or two higher than I was used to, or because there were more buildings shielding me from the winds, or more traffic fumes – the famous London smog. London is hardly Las Vegas but it felt overwhelming to me; muggy, hypnotically brighter and louder, the puddles in the road gleaming with rainbows of oily colour which were unseemly somehow, and wave after wave of people stampeding down the pavement so I could never quite walk in a straight line. Reading, I discovered, was a different type of pastime in London. People read on the move: magazines, newspapers, even books!

They read as they were walking on pavements, travelling on escalators and – very carelessly – while crossing roads. I never considered reading to be an ambulatory activity until I moved to London. I still live in the capital and have come to love its quirks: the people so desperate to read they walk into lamp posts, the bright red sign that warns 'Do Not Feed the Pigeons' which has been vandalised by someone who has written over the word 'Pigeons' with 'Tories', the constant feeling of being told off by unseen dictators via loudspeaker – 'Do not cross the yellow line: stand back from the platform edge' and 'Do not stand on the left of the escalator: walk on the left and stand on the right'. Jeez, there are so many rules! Back then, it was all quite alien to me. I think, as much as I was excited to move to the 'Big Smoke' and climb up a rung on the career ladder, there was still a feeling of unease because I associated the city with those July terror attacks. I hoped it wouldn't last.

As a new arrival in London, I was entitled to move into NHS accommodation – the place near the prison, asylum and graveyard which would make the perfect horror movie. The building was practically derelict and very unkempt and I couldn't believe that the people who were helping to save lives in the hospital, such as the nurses, were living there. It was like a Soviet Gulag camp: smashed windows, mouse droppings in the shared kitchen cupboards, barbed-wire fences. Because I also had to walk through a pretty rough housing estate to get to my accommodation I was terrified of having to return after dark. I might be having a coffee with a friend one day and notice the sun starting to set so I'd jump up and run off like Cinderella, trotting down the High Street on foot to get to the Gulag before sundown.

Early nights were probably for the best anyway. At the Metropolitan the system was different from what I'd been used to. We APTs had to be in for seven a.m. and the post-mortems started at about seven thirty as the pathologist, Dr Singh, headed to one mortuary after another, carrying out as many cases as he could. I was happy to get out of the Gulag as early as possible every morning anyway, but on my first day I got a bit lost wandering round the hospital complex. When I did arrive it was slightly later than planned.

'What the . . . ?' I exclaimed, on entering that first day. I'd been shown into a small utility room containing a washer, a dryer and several shelves which held what I assumed were clean scrubs, but they weren't folded or in any particular size order. There was a pile of them on the floor so I assumed they were the dirty ones.

The manager, Danny, said, 'We've got the cases out and ready so just get some scrubs that fit and crack on.'

Easier said than done, I thought, as I eyed up the mismatched pile (some were green, some were blue), but I managed to dig out some coordinating 'smalls' and some size 5 wellington boots. It was clear there was no laundry collection service here and the APTs were 'responsible' for their own washing and drying. As the only female on the team I was certain this was to become my job from now on.

On entering the autopsy room I again exclaimed 'What the . . . ?' There were six post-mortem tables in this new place and every single one of them was occupied. That seemed like a lot of cases, certainly more than I was used to at the Municipal Mortuary, but there were to be three technicians working so it wasn't too bad. I was just perplexed that everything was in full swing so early in the morning: all the patients were already open, in that they'd each had their sternum removed and their internal organs were glistening under the multitude of lights on the huge PM room ceiling. It was Chris, the assistant manager, who'd dashed through all the cases, whizzing through the process of making the incisions and removing the sterna only, his bald head also glistening under the lights as he moved deftly.

'Right, here's what we're gonna do,' he said to me author-itatively as Ryan entered the PM room with the pathologist right behind him. 'You've been doing the Y-incision in the last place, haven't you? Well, we do the I-incision here and it has to be quite low down so the family can't see it. For today I'm doing all the incisions because I need Ryan to show you something else we do different.'

I nodded my head. Basically, the pathologist was already there and ready to start, so Chris didn't have time to fanny about with me right now making slow, unfamiliar incisions, i.e. straight lines.

'Ryan, go over there with Carla and show her the method,' Chris shouted as he pointed with a bloody PM40 to a male patient on the first table with not only his sternum but also his bowels removed.

I was getting nervous. What 'method'? Why all the mili-tary orders? I hadn't even had a cup of coffee yet.

Ryan, obviously used to Chris's curt manner, took me over to the first patient in a relaxed way and said, 'Basically, we take the organs out in blocks here so I think Chris wants you to practise doing that on all these cases. I'll show you it so that the doc can crack on with mine, then you can do the other five.'

'So you mean you use the en bloc method of Ghon, rather

than the en masse method of Letulle, usually incorrectly referred to as the Rokitansky Method?' I said, like a total smart-arse. 'And you think you need to teach me that?' I even pulled my visor down and looked over the top of it at him like an annoyed school teacher.

He obviously knew the mechanics of their system but perhaps not the history behind it. He looked at me, surprised that I did. 'OK – go ahead.'

'Do you want the neck and tongue?'

'Nah. I'll go and start on the next one.'

It's true that we commonly took out all of the organs en masse at the Municipal Mortuary but I had worked at other mortuaries, sometimes filling in for people off sick, sometimes training, and, of course, there was the mass fatality incident in London. I was used to varying my methods.

The fact that the pathologist didn't want the neck and tongue removed made this very simple for me. I bent down over the deceased with my trusty PM40 at the ready and sliced across the oesophagus and trachea at the level of the clavicles. Then I carried out my usual scooping check behind the lungs: *slap*, the left one was unattached; *slap*, the right one was unattached. All I then had to do was sever the oesophagus, trachea and aorta beneath the lungs and above the diaphragm and there it was: the cardiorespiratory block or 'pluck'. This contained only those organs necessary for respiration – the lungs and, of course, the heart – which were within what is known as the mediastinum: the central compartment of the thoracic cavity. It allowed the pathologist immediately to focus on the dissection of the heart – the most important organ in terms of cause of death – without waiting for the rest of the viscera to be removed. Statistics vary, but in general coronary heart disease (CHD) leading to heart attacks and heart failure is the main cause of death both in the UK and worldwide. Yet experts say that most cases of premature death from heart disease are completely preventable. Smoking, being overweight, having high blood pressure and/or high cholesterol, heavy drinking and physical inactivity are all key risk factors.

Why don't we take the heart more seriously, as a culture? This precious organ is literally the epicentre of our physiological existence and is also symbolically so important. The Ancient Egyptians believed that the heart and not the brain was the source of wisdom in humans (as well as the soul, the personality, the emotions and memories) and it was therefore one of the only organs left in situ during the mummification process. In the fourth century BC the heart was identified by the Greek philosopher Aristotle as the most important organ in the body, 'a three-chambered repository that was the seat of vitality, reason and intelligence'. However, in the second century AD our Mel Gibson of Medicine, Galen, considered the heart to be most closely related to the soul (as we do today), and some of my favourite historical quotes on the heart's function come from him. 'The heart is hard flesh, not easily injured,' he said. 'In hardness, tension, general strength, and resistance to injury, the fibres of the heart far surpass all others, for no other instrument performs such continuous, hard work as the heart.' I like to think of this 'hard work' as being emotional as well as physical. I'm certain everyone reading this will have had their heart take an absolute battering at some point in their romantic lives, but of course the pain does go away – eventually – and the heart recovers.

In the twelfth century, the popularity of medieval courtly love caused another switch in opinion and cemented the connections between the anatomical heart, the heart shape that we now see on all our Valentine cards (which is called a 'cardioid' in geometry) and the idea of romantic love. The heart was used to symbolise this courtly love on banners and shields; then, despite the Church attempting to monopolise the symbol for their images of the Immaculate Heart of Mary and the Sacred Heart of Jesus, the heart penetrated further into the public domain when, around 1480, it was chosen to represent one of the suits of cards.*

I held at least one human heart in my hand nearly every single day of my life as an APT, and this day was no different. Washed clean beneath running tap water, its thick dark blood clots removed and swirling down the plughole so it was ready for the pathologist to dissect, this organ was still a miracle to me, no matter how familiar the process. The fact that it did look like the cardioid shape on a Valentine card; the fact that it fitted in my hand yet contained the electrical impulses necessary to keep humans twice my size alive; the fact that it could stop beating and start again in certain circumstances – all of those things ran through my mind each time I held one, and I felt I could hear my own heart beat louder in recognition of its power. In the cartoon from the 1980s, He-Man used to hold his sword aloft and shout 'By the power of Greyskull!' and light would flow from the sword and change him. I wanted to do the same thing: I felt like, if I held

---

* I find it quite humorous that the Church ever did want to 'own' the heart as a sort of trademark given that another explanation for its shape is fairly risqué: the cardioid represents genitals. The right way up it represents the vulva, and upside down, the testicles.

a heart high above my head, beams of light like those from the Sacred Heart would radiate from it and I could shout, 'I have the powwwweeer!'

I obviously didn't do that.

I'm not the only one who understands the heart's majesty. Nowadays, at the museum, I teach people to preserve organs in glass jars using the same method I would with the rest of the collection. I always give a choice of kidneys or hearts and it's inevitably the hearts people want to preserve or 'pot'. They poke them tentatively with gloved fingers, pore over them (usually working in twos), and exchange them when they're finished. 'Here, have my heart, darling,' and so on.

The heart is a fragile yet potent item. In some ways, it's just as Galen said, resilient because 'no other instrument performs such continuous, hard work'. But in other ways, the heart can be as fragile as a dried flower and just as easily crushed.

I must have stood there thinking for far too long because Chris suddenly shouted to me, 'Get a move on, girl – we need to race and see who can open the bodies the quickest. The loser buys everyone lunch.'

Since there were six post-mortem tables in this new place – much larger than my last – we'd autopsy up to five or six adults a day on a rota system, and there was no way I was getting out of autopsying bariatric bodies here: at the Metropolitan I had no special treatment due to my size. Each week, a specific APT was assigned to office work only, a specific one to perinatal (baby) PMs only, and the other two or three APTs would handle the rest. As there were a few of us, all very experienced, the cases could all be finished by ten a.m. I was not used to that. At the Municipal Mortuary I was used to two autopsies and their paperwork taking us right up to lunchtime around one p.m. I was used to undertakers arriving throughout the afternoon to bring in cases from the outside or to collect decedents for funeral homes. As I had been 'a trainee' there, it had been my job to answer the ringing doorbell and become proficient at dealing with the paperwork. I did it so often I developed a Pavlovian response to any type of 'ding-dong' noise.* Now that there was always someone designated as the office worker here, I didn't have to answer so frequently, and we had an intercom rather than a doorbell.

The situation was inevitably going to feel different for a while. One thing I found particular to London (or perhaps just my new mortuary) was the use of the word 'cunt'. Up north, that word is like 'Voldemort' – something that shouldn't be said out loud. If you used it in an argument the whole room would go quiet. At the Metropolitan it was used like punctuation, and peppered nearly every sentence: 'Make me a cuppa tea, you cunt' or 'Go and measure the bodies, you cunt'. Here a cunt, there a cunt, everywhere a cunt, cunt.

In that place I couldn't move for cunts.

I don't know what it's like to have children, but I think my experience working at the Metropolitan gave me an idea of how it could be. I'd known it would be a male team, but in contrast to the mixed-gender situation at the temporary

---

* This became hilariously evident to friends of mine when we were in restaurants that announce that hot food is ready to be served by ringing a bell on the dumb waiter. Every single time the bell went I'd jump out of my seat. It took *ages* for me to repress that response once I'd left the Municipal Mortuary.

mortuary for 7/7, this place had a different dynamic. There was a lot of testosterone in one small place. Of the more junior ATPs, the more evolved Josh brought some welcome sensitivity and common sense into the environment, but Ryan was more outwardly confident. Although I thought of them as the Terror Trio (I excluded Josh), all four men were either related or very close family friends who'd known each other for years. As a result, they had a bond with each other that left me feeling as though I was on the outside, looking in.

I don't think I'd ever been in such a close-knit situation with so many men in my life, and, given that I had undergone such a dramatic upheaval, the problems that would eventually occur were inevitable. I was too vulnerable. Normally fairly tough, among these men I was like a fragile flower; it just wasn't the right situation for me to be in. For that reason, when I look back on the time I spent with the 'boisterous' boys at the Metropolitan, I try to see the best in it despite all their escapades. However, they were constantly scrapping and joking and their mock insults extended to practically everyone, whether inside the team or out.

There was an undertaker who would come to the department every now and again and he had a deformed hand. Two of my colleagues would carry on a conversation with him, acting as normally as possible, yet all the while trying slyly to squeeze the word 'hand' in, like some sort of dare, to see who could do it the most.

'Let me give you a *hand* with that,' said one, exaggerating the word.

'Nah, I'm sure he can *hand*le it,' said the other, with a wink.

'Well, if you change your mind we'll be all *hand*s on deck,' replied the first.

I knew the undertaker could tell they were making fun of him and chose to ignore their remarks and rise above it, but it can't have been easy to be on the receiving end of a prank like this. I was unhappy, not necessarily with the job but with the accommodation difficulties, the upheaval and the general atmosphere. It was a cocktail of negativity. Perhaps I *was* living above an Indian burial ground after all? A month or two after my arrival I managed to find myself a cheap room in a shared house just by the tube station and ten minutes' walk from the mortuary. Saying goodbye to the Gulag was a much-needed boost, but I was still living with strangers – forced to by London prices. After previously having my own little Rose Cottage it felt like a huge step down.

A certain level of strength is something we are all born with, and then, as we grow, we learn to be stronger. I'll freely admit I did not feel strong at that time. Alone and lonely, working hard from seven a.m. to keep the negative thoughts at bay and attending the gym every night to avoid going back to a house of people I didn't know, I was becoming fatigued. Even my long-distance boyfriend was noticing my lack of enthusiasm and energy for nightly phone calls. Carrying out four to five adult autopsies and dealing with riotous men daily was physically draining but it didn't distract me from exercise. I'd remove my scrubs at the end of the long day, throw them into the washing machine with the others and change into my shorts and vest for yet more physical exertion at the gym. But for some reason, that didn't stop one of them from commenting that I was gaining weight. 'You go to the gym a lot but by the size of you, you must be going home and stuffing your face!' he said to me one day. Bear in mind he was no oil painting himself and in no position to point fingers, his comments made me paranoid, made me question myself. Was I gaining weight? I couldn't understand how it was possible – I was barely ever sitting down and I barely had time to eat. So I started going to the gym *twice* a day, still attending my usual leisure centre in the evenings but fitting in forty-five minutes at the hospital gym at lunch, too.

The weight gain, thankfully, was temporary – a simple side effect of my new contraceptive pill. The barbed comments from my colleagues, however, were not. They were either directed at me, at each other, or to visitors coming in. It was exhausting trying to keep an eye on them or work out how or what they would do next. Some afternoons, their morning antics must have fatigued them because one might pull the office blinds down and actually take a nap. Relief would wash over me; in the silence, I'd feel like a parent who could finally relax. I'd make a cup of tea and study for my Diploma, dealing with any visitors as they arrived, 'shushing' them and closing the door of the office quietly behind me as I did so, in order to make sure the sleeper did not wake up.

When they finally did, towards the end of our day, about three p.m., I'd wander into the PM room, despite all our cases being completed and the room having been cleaned. I'd go on tidiness detail: bleach the scalpel handles, use forceps to pull old hair from the drains, organise drawers and trays, wash all our scrubs in the washing machine, fold the ones that had been washed and dried then put them all in size-order, colour-coordinated piles. *Anything* to just be doing something. If there really was nothing to do I'd wander away from them to the place where we carried out viewings and let the silence wash over me like an elixir.

I spent a lot of time alone in that mortuary.

I'm not completely socially inept, of course, and I did find time to chat with visitors, particularly the newer undertakers who came to collect the deceased and convey them to various funeral homes. And I was meeting other APTs every Thursday afternoon when I attended the lectures for my Diploma course. I even saw a few of those colleagues socially – just for a drink or a bite to eat, nothing romantic; just trying to make friends. To me, it didn't seem like an odd thing to accept a night out with a person my own age in the same field of work, no matter what their gender, especially considering this was a new city for me and I didn't know anyone. But nearly all undertakers and APTs at that time were male, and who knows, maybe my socialising rubbed up the team at the Metropolitan the wrong way? Maybe they thought I was going further despite having a boyfriend up north, and that explains what I felt was disrespect towards me? But I wasn't after anyone's heart – or any other part of their anatomy. I tried to keep that interest strictly in the post-mortem room! The long-distance relationship with my northern boyfriend was ending and I needed no further complications down south. I didn't even have the basics yet: a home I wanted to live in, a good girl friend, a decent hairdresser and a favourite coffee shop. I was simply a functioning mortician who lived for work – lived for the dead and the dead only. I began to relish being alone and pulled even further away from the boys. I listened to music as I worked; these were patients who deserved care and attention to detail and music helped me relax and focus on my tasks, limiting any mistakes. I didn't want to lose a finger.

Another thing I didn't want to lose was my heart. But when feeling so vulnerable and lonely, it was inevitable that

I'd project that on to someone – the one person in the group who was mentoring me, showing me some kindness and highlighting a sensitive side. Josh, the youngest of the APTs, became the one and only person there I actually wanted to talk to. How much did I *really* like him? I'm still not sure. Perhaps I simply disliked the others so much he was the best option for companionship and camaraderie: there seemed to be an inverse correlation between how little I began to like the Terror Trio and how much I began to like Josh. With his floppy brown hair and gentle nature he was an inevitable magnet for someone who was hurting; someone like me. It was a closeness and friendship I needed there and then, and it went a long way towards comforting me.

Often, when the Terror Trio were asleep or out and the day's work was all done, Josh and I would sit and watch films together while we waited for the mortuary intercom to buzz.

'What? You've never seen *Labyrinth*?' he exclaimed, during one of our conversations, then acted out what I assumed was a pivotal scene: 'I move the stars for no one!'

I looked at him totally blankly.

'Right, that's it, I'm bringing it in tomorrow,' he threatened – and he did. We sat side by side in the quiet office with the blinds drawn and the others dozing around us, knowing we'd be interrupted by an undertaker or two to collect a patient but that it wouldn't wake them – we'd deal with that ourselves using the pause button. Then sometimes, when spending time with him, I began to wish that life had a pause button; that we could keep talking and be left in peace with everything around us not existing just for a short while.

I suppose my feelings blossomed too much, not like a rose but like the *Ipomoea alba*, the moonflower, which only blooms at night – during the wrong time, a dark time. Their petals close when they eventually feel the sun. Given that Josh had been with his girlfriend for many years and I was rebounding, it was not a safe or healthy situation for me. I realised I needed to go off and 'feel the sun', to make London a happy home, but perhaps based somewhere else. I began to consider removing the heart of my problems and leaving, but even though there was never anything romantic between Josh and me, I will always be grateful for his friendship when I needed it the most.

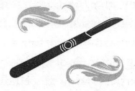

Sometimes APTs need to remove the heart of a person who doesn't need a post-mortem and is an organ donor. In this particular situation, when a patient is already deceased, the heart can't be transplanted fully into a live patient who needs a whole heart: that can only occur when the donor is on life support. Basically, their body must be functioning but they will inevitably be what is known as 'brain stem dead'. The family will make a decision to turn off the life support machine at a particular time, giving the recipient and surgeons a chance to prepare for the intricate procedure with a fresh heart. Instead, when the deceased has been dead a short while and received into a mortuary, the valves specifically can be removed for implanting into patients who may need valve repair or replacement. When human donor valves are used for this purpose they're called homografts, but sometimes mechanical valves and even pig or cow heart valves can be used. This procedure, however, has to take place within forty-eight hours after death, as long as the deceased has been refrigerated within six hours of death. If no refrigeration has occurred, the removal must be within twelve hours. As long as we can remove the whole heart in time and pack it correctly, then courier it to the relevant tissue bank, a living patient can reap the benefits of the valves from the dead heart.

Chris was experienced in heart retrievals and showed me how to do it one day, in an unusual fit of patient mentoring. To be fair, for all his faults he was the most knowledgeable APT at the Metropolitan and the most active PM-wise. He began by explaining that the instruments we were to use were set aside for this purpose only. After handing me the specific PM40, he said, 'You can go ahead and do the cut as usual,' so I cracked on with the straight incision then removed the sternum and ribs with the designated rib shears.

'I'll take over now,' he said, but he didn't take the PM40 from me once I'd finished. Instead, he opened a dedicated, single-use heart retrieval kit which had been provided by NHS Blood and Transplant Services (NHSBT) specifically for this point where the donor deceased had been opened. This was to minimise the risk of cross-contamination from the outside of the body.

'Right,' he continued authoritatively, talking me through his actions, 'this is very different to removing the cardiorespiratory block. What you need to do is use these disposable scissors to cut the pericardium, being careful not to touch the lungs or anything else with the tip of them.'

The pericardium, also known as the heart sac, is a

double-layered serous and fibrous membrane that surrounds the heart and contains some fluid so that the beating organ within pulses across it repeatedly with ease. It protects the heart from infection and lubricates it.

Chris gently sliced through the membrane and there in all its usual glory was the distinctive striated muscle of the heart.

'Now, with this disposable scalpel we need to cut the vessels at the top of the heart as high up as we can to give NHSBT as much as possible to work with.' He did so, and soon was holding aloft the heart in what had now become a familiar gesture. He didn't change into He-Man though.

'Right, grab them two swabs and take a swipe at two different areas of the cardiac tissue – I won't move my hands.' I did so, labelled them, and laid them gently down. This was to ensure the heart could be checked for infection at NHSBT.

'Now we can rinse it in Hartmann's solution,' he said, to which I responded incredulously, '*Heart*man's solution – are you serious?'

He got the joke. 'Hahaha. Nah, it's just an aptly named infusion which closely resembles blood. It's what you get in a drip.'

'Ah.' I realised what he meant. Hartmann's solution is an isotonic fluid that was created by US paediatrician A. F. Hartmann, who was born in 1898. It's so closely isotonic with blood – that is, it's got the same osmotic or 'liquid' pressure – that it's usually intended for intravenous administration via a hospital drip, replacing body fluid and mineral salts that may be lost for a variety of medical reasons. In this instance, it would keep the heart stable for transport.

After rinsing, the precious organ was placed in a single-use plastic bag and then Chris handed me a polystyrene box for it to go in with the bacterial swabs and a kilogram of ice to be stuffed in around it.

'There you go,' he said. 'Get packing.'

It just so happened that later that evening I found myself packing again, this time my belongings ... but things were actually looking up and I wasn't packing to move far. One of my housemates, Mal, who rented the largest room of our three-bed house, had moved out. I'd met a friend, a lawyer named Denise, at my Amnesty International meetings and she needed a new place to live so I moved to the bigger room and she moved into my old one. Suddenly I was feeling more settled. I was living with someone I considered a friend, I was meeting other APTs at my course, and I'd even learned a new skill that day.

My life began to feel like it was coming together.

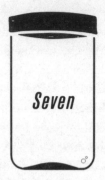

Seven

Abdominal Block: 'Pickled Punks'

Bruises on the fruit.
Tender age in bloom.

—*Nirvana, 'In Bloom'*

The anatomical displays at Victorian medical museums and carnival freak shows which I alluded to earlier consisted of a melange of curios: incredible examples of 'mermaids', which were actually composites of monkey and fish skeletons, and, of course, bearded or tattooed ladies, the proverbial Strongman and individuals in the unfortunate position of having unusual deformities. In addition to these clichés, genuine human tissue specimens had laymen in awe, as they were preserved examples of their own, hitherto unseen, body parts. Those titillating female Anatomical Venuses, and smaller wax moulages of body parts, also had the general public attending these carnivals in droves. However, one of the biggest draws was the 'pickled punks', an old carny term for preserved whole baby specimens. Of course, we never use the term 'pickled punks' in a contemporary museum setting because it's anachronistic and unethical. Yet despite the more modern way in which they are educationally referenced and displayed – as foetal or perinatal specimens – they still remain contentious and create a huge divide in opinion on the ethics of display.

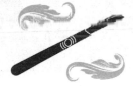

The different methods of organ removal used in mortuaries meant that after the cardiorespiratory block had been extracted the APT would usually move on to the coeliac block – the pluck of organs containing the stomach, pancreas, liver and spleen. Then the genitourinary block containing the kidneys, adrenals, bladder and genital organs would be removed.

I'll never forget the first time I saw the uterus and ovaries of a normal, albeit deceased, woman during my early training. 'That's *it*?' I'd shouted furiously, causing the heads of the other APTs and doctors in the room to turn towards me. I couldn't believe how small they all were! After all the years of menstrual cramps and all the discomfort I'd experienced due to PMT, I imagined the uterus to be a bright red demonic entity covered in spikes which would bare its teeth at me as I attempted to remove it. Instead, it resembled a little pink plum, and the ovaries two matching fleshy almonds. They looked so harmless. I was shocked that something that insipid could cause so much woe! Of course, I (begrudgingly) got used to the uniformity of size and colour of these organs until the first time the uterus I exposed really was a lot larger than it was supposed to be and I had to alert the pathologist.

'Doc, can you come and take a look at this?' I'd asked, unsure how to proceed.

He came over and palpated the organ before making a careful, long incision to reveal a tiny, angelic baby nestled inside the dead woman's uterus. It was exactly like the final reveal of what Joanna Ebenstein described as the 'tranquil foetus curled in the womb of the wax Anatomical Venuses of old', their sex specifically used as a tool to teach students about the creation, development and even destruction of life.

The womb can also be a tomb.

Mortuary work, of course, involves the autopsy and dissection of foetuses and newborns, because it is a sad truth that babies die too, whether in utero, during birth or a short time after. Culturally, we don't like to consider this: people don't want to think about the miniature 'dolls' house' set of autopsy tools reserved specifically for the perinatal bench, or the tiny rectangular coffins and petite plastic body bags mortuaries have to purchase in bulk. The coffins in particular, which come in an Ikea flat-pack-style cardboard, are a strange hybrid: on the one hand, a repository for the remains of someone's dead child, on the other, a *possible* place to store shoes. Fears about the processes of neo- or perinatal autopsies abound because there is a natural, maternal sense of horror at the idea of such a delicate and innocent human being under-going the ordeal.

But it *is* necessary.

For the most part, at the Metropolitan, the perinatal autop-sies were not ordered by the Coroner but consented to by the parents. About 15 to 25 per cent of recognised pregnancies will end in a miscarriage and more than 80 per cent of miscarriages occur within the first three months of pregnancy. The shocked and devastated parents, when approached for their consent, usually agreed to (or often even independently requested) a post-mortem because they wanted answers. Was there some-thing that caused the baby's death that they could avoid doing in the next pregnancy? Was there a genetic issue that needed treatment to ensure successful future pregnancies?

The first time I carried out an autopsy on a baby was at the Metropolitan, and it was a completely different process from what I was used to with adults. I welcomed learning this new skill in order to develop as an APT, and thankfully, of all the men there who could have been my mentor, it was Josh that I shadowed. He was a good buffer for the shock of seeing a dead baby laid out for autopsy for the first time: no teasing, no cleverness; just patience. And seeing a deceased child about to be eviscerated, no matter what age it is, is a shock, even for someone like myself who'd worked with the dead for over three years at this point and seen pretty much everything.

The first baby we autopsied together was a male who had passed away in utero, meaning he wasn't old enough to resemble a baby. At around seventeen to eighteen weeks' ges-tation, his skin was delicate (or 'friable') and very red rather than pink because it was macerated, which means he had been soaking and softening in the live mother's amniotic fluid after his death. (This tissue degeneration arises because of autolytic enzymes, just like adults have when they die, but because the fluid is a sterile solution there is no bacterial action and therefore no 'proper' decomposition.) Physically, his proportions were not the same as a full-term baby. His head-to-body ratio was more consistent with an adult's, and the limbs were long and lithe, not chubby and peachy like a sweet-smelling newborn. As a result, he looked like a small adult who'd been scalded, some of the skin peeling off due to the maceration. He also had a slightly reptilian or alien appearance. As unusual as he looked in some respects, he was recognisably human: there were minuscule pale eyelashes around the closed eyes – eyes that hadn't opened yet and never would – and there were tiny fingers which unbelievably already had fingernails the size of pinheads. He was still clearly a little miracle. I've never been maternal but I recognised it as a special thing, this child, and I didn't like the way the perinatal pathologist picked him up by his feet and dropped him on to the weighing scales, as though she was a fishmonger with a sea bass. Was this the way all perinatal pathologists did it? I didn't know – I didn't know anything about the procedure at this point and was feeling confused as the doctor began to dictate and Josh took notes.

The world of the perinatal post-mortem involves some unfamiliar vocabulary. For the first time I was hearing words like 'vernix' and 'lanugo': vernix is the white, waxy substance you see coating newborns (usually on TV, unless your hobby is hanging around maternity wards), and lanugo is the fine downy hair that develops on foetuses in the womb at about five months and sheds into the amniotic fluid at around seven or eight months. Wait, there's more: because the foetus consumes amniotic fluid for nourishment it also eats the shedded lanugo hair, and this partly makes up the baby's meconium – that's their first poo.

What crazy new world was this? I already thought babies were freaky alive – I couldn't hold them or feed them as I really didn't have any experience with them, coming from a small family, and when I was out and about I didn't want to hear or smell them – but I was discovering they were even more complicated in death.

Thankfully, Josh talked me through the process as I watched, rapt. During a perinatal autopsy, after the weight and height of the tiny cadaver have been recorded to determine the exact gestation, it is the perinatal pathologist who carries out the delicate dissection, not us. We, the APTs, stand by to record measurements, hand over specific tools and help to place minuscule tissue samples into various pots and cassettes. The perinatal pathologists alone are familiar with the organs of a foetus, or neonate, which are so small the tissues are visually barely distinguishable from one another. In fact, we technicians aren't even required to open the head as we would with adult cases. The pathologists can reflect the thin scalp skin back themselves then cut through the delicate skull bones with scissors. A saw is not needed on such fragile skull cartilage which has not yet had the chance to ossify into proper bone, particularly the soft open area at the top, the fontanelle.

The main tasks we perform are taking notes and suspending the brain in formalin* to 'fix' it for about a week before

---

* Formalin is the aqueous solution used in the preservation of tissue, not formaldehyde, which is a gas. Formalin is formaldehyde distributed through water, and it's used in mortuaries, histology labs, etc.

it can be examined – it's much too soft at this stage to be dissected by the pathologist, and I can really only describe it as delicate pink blancmange which barely has the markings of the brain images we are so familiar with. The other task we have is to reconstruct the tiny cadaver in the event that the parents would like to view their child, and of course we would let them do so as soon as physically possible.

'I don't understand it, Josh,' I said, after that first perinatal autopsy during which I'd done nothing but watch and ask a million questions. 'How can the parents see their baby this afternoon if the head is sliced open and the brain is meant to stay over there for a week?' I pointed to a labelled Tupperware pot in which the delicate pale mass was submerged in fluid on a dedicated 'brain shelf' among countless others.

'We don't need the brain to be in the head,' Josh explained patiently as he removed a small piece of cotton wool from a large roll, formed it into a ball roughly the size of the pink cerebral tissue that had been removed, and placed it delicately into the empty skull.

It was starting to make sense but I still had a query: 'But if we stitch that up now we'll have to unstitch it to put the brain back in next week, won't we? Then stitch it again? It'll look messy.'

Ever patient, Josh simply reached for some cyanoacrylate, or 'superglue' – something I was about to learn is the mortician's best-kept secret, and which really earns its name – and said, 'We can't stitch this. Look, it's too friable.' He was right. It was like the skin of a recently burned victim; it would tear too easily. Instead, I watched, fascinated, as he neatly folded the edges of the doctor's incision so they were perfectly straight, delicately lay a trail of glue along the skin of one incision, then pressed the other edge against it, holding for a few seconds.

The line that joined the two pieces of scalp together was as thin as a hair and barely noticeable. I looked at him, impressed.

There wasn't much time for admiration, though, because the glue dried quickly and he gently turned the baby over on to his back to reveal the empty thoracic cavity.

'Right – your turn.'

OK, the first problem here was that lying on the small dissection board I had a tiny pile of miniature organs and tissues which all looked the same anaemic pink. They needed to go back into the baby and an adult viscera bag was obviously not the way to do it. That's when I spied the clingfilm. I reached for it and Josh nodded his approval at my correct assumption. I removed a piece of the awkward clingy plastic, scraped the organs and tissues gently on to it with a small blade, then wrapped it up into a neat package which fitted into the cavity perfectly. Then, taking the superglue, I attempted the same technique as Josh. He had made it look effortless. It was actually as fiddly as hell but I got there in the end, the miniature torso now intact with a little line down the middle no wider than a piece of embroidery thread. I felt a flush of pride when I saw him smile at my efforts, but as usual there was no time for revelling in small achievements. We were already moving on to the next task.

'Right, we'd better get him dressed and set up for viewing.'

At first, I hadn't understood what Josh meant when he said we had to 'dress' the first Lilliputian cadaver I'd ever encountered. Surely clothes were not made for babies so small that they wouldn't survive outside the womb. Did we buy dolls' clothes, perhaps? I came to learn that volunteers actually knitted miniature garments in pink and blue, usually hats and cardigans, specifically for these tiny viewings. The hats in particular were welcome because they helped to humanise the odd-looking little corpses and hide the incisions at the back, no matter how neatly they had been reconstructed.

As the only female on the team here, I seemed to become the go-to girl for perinatal viewings arranged by the Bereavement Service's head officer. I found that I liked the job of carrying them out: I cared that the child was dressed correctly and that any toys or photographs the parents had requested to be placed in the small crib were there as they should be. I got used to the unfamiliar perinatal world and I felt like I could communicate with these devastated parents at such a difficult time much more appropriately than the Terror Trio could. Plus, it gave me more tasks to do in the afternoon to keep me away from the rest of the team. Often, Josh would come and help, and that was fine – he was sensitive to the parents' needs in the same way I was. What with the baby viewings and studying for my Diploma I began to feel like I had my own specific purposes at this mortuary and they didn't really involve spending a lot of time with the others.

Which suited me just fine.

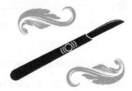

Why is it that baby viewings require such a delicate touch? It may seem like a stupidly obvious question since they're babies and 'their death is a shock' so it's incredibly sad, but that can apply to many decedents. Lots of people lose a loved one suddenly, someone they may have been close to for years such as a sibling, a parent, a best friend. They too deserve the same amount of care and attention. Yet there is a good reason why there is more sensitivity towards baby viewings. Perhaps it the sadness is about a life which never had the chance to start; the hopes for a child and their innocence.

In the UK in the late 1990s, something called the organ retention scandal or Alder Hey scandal occurred. It began when a bereaved mother learned that her child's heart had been kept for testing at a Bristol hospital without her knowledge (meaning she had unwittingly buried her child incomplete). There was then an investigation in which it transpired the same type of organ retention occurred at Alder Hey Hospital in Liverpool, not far from where I'd been working. Further investigations uncovered another two hundred or so hospitals and teaching facilities which routinely retained organs, despite parents not being aware of it, simply because it wasn't specifically stipulated in the Human Tissue Act of 1961 that their permission needed to be sought. The public was outraged, and the media didn't help the sensitive situation, writing articles under head-lines such as 'Ghoulish Malpractice!' and 'Return of the Body Snatchers!' In truth, nothing illegal had occurred, except in the case of one dodgy pathologist who went by the gothic horror name Dr Dick van Velzen. He was based at Alder Hey, which meant a lot of the focus ended up on that hospital – which is why the scandal is often referred to as 'Alder Hey' for short. An organisation of bereaved par-ents demanded a change to the law and the Human Tissue

Authority was eventually formed in the UK in 2005. Their job was to ensure that 'informed consent' for any organ retention was obtained from next of kin, and to govern the use of human tissue for post-mortems, public display, some transplants and more. This is why we had to treat baby viewings carefully, despite the fact that most parents were happy to discuss their babies' autopsies and routinely agreed to tissue retention. It seems that, for some people, the stigma of the 1990s scandal hasn't left when it comes to deceased babies, but it also seems that neither has the anxiety or dread of being buried 'incomplete' in some way, mirroring those fears of cadaver dissection from the past.

This has left us with a skewed vision of perinatal autopsies and medical specimens such as those on the shelves of my museum, despite the fact we don't treat them like the pickled punks of old. Why are most people more sensitive about them than they are with adult specimens? Perhaps babies floating in preservative fluid or laid out on an autopsy table, completely whole, are more recognisably human with their tiny eyelashes, fingers and toes? Or is it the idea of an innocent wasted life that makes some people more sensitive to deceased babies in general? Some feel that exhibiting these specimens in museums is traumatic to those who have suffered a miscarriage or stillbirth. But then what of the female pathologists, police personnel, social workers and others who have experienced these traumas in their personal lives as well as in their careers? Do they stop working? Does everything come to a standstill?

I was about to discover that no, it does not. Life goes on.

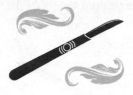

In one way my life was definitely moving on. I saw a job advertised for a Senior APT in another London mortuary, St Martin's Hospital, which I could apply for now that I was a Diploma-holding technician. I was as highly qualified as an APT could be, on paper. My interview again involved a panel of four people but it was something I'd become used to and I gave it my all. I was confident and capable, and, more importantly, I was beginning to shake off the negativity of the past year. After more than five years I was experienced in embalming as well as all aspects of mortuary work and nearly every post-mortem possible: Coronial, hospital, forensic, perinatal. The only thing I'd never experienced enough of were autopsies of individuals designated High Risk; that is, decedents with a known infectious disease, intravenous drug users, and people who have been exposed to dangerous chemicals or radiation. Such 'High Risk' autopsies could only be performed by a Senior APT.

I needed that experience, and I needed to get out of the hospital I was working in. I was a good APT but I wanted to be great, and St Martin's was one of the best places to learn. My enthusiasm and hunger for the challenge must have been very obvious during the interview and my CV must have backed up my claims of competence because I hadn't even left the hospital grounds when one of the interviewers called my mobile phone.

I'd done it – I was offered the job. I literally skipped out of the hospital gate.

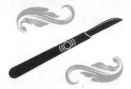

What a contrasting experience St Martin's was! It was hectic in a whole different way to the last place. There I had only been occupied when I chose to keep myself occupied. Here I had no choice: I was constantly buzzing around the mortuary like a *Calliphora vomitoria* (that's the scientific terminology for a blue-arsed fly). It was the busiest, most productive mortuary I'd ever been in. And talk about extremes: I'd gone from a team of four boys to a team of five girls which was actually about to become six as there was a new trainee starting, so *seven* including me. So much testosterone in an enclosed environment had been a problem in the last place; how would I fare with a massive cocktail of oestrogen?

Time would tell.

At least the overall manager of the facility who popped in now and again, Juan, was male and able to add a bit of masculinity to the proceedings. I had met him before at the 7/7 facility and I liked him. He was ambitious and inspiring, gentle and encouraging, but tough when he needed to be. I was happy to be working with him.

The first day I started there I tried to act as comfortable as possible even though I was crazy nervous – a year of working with four men who resembled The Young Ones does that to a girl. But, newly single and ready to mingle, it was nice to be part of a gaggle of girls and in a totally different environment. It was a change I sorely needed.

As we sat down that first morning to introduce ourselves over coffee I spotted a copy of *Maxim* magazine in the office next to the computer. '*Maxim*? Isn't that a bloke's magazine? It can't be Juan's, can it?' I said, with a wink.

The girls laughed, and Sharon, the other Senior APT and my closest colleague, replied, 'Nah, we bought it because it's got a big feature on the funeral directors we work closely with: Anderson Morgan Funeral Service in South London.'

'Ah,' I said, as I flicked through the magazine with interest, and sure enough there were about six pages dedicated to Anderson Morgan. It was a very well-known family-run establishment which had been the focus of a TV show and had carried out some high-profile funerals.

I stopped, mid-flick, to focus on a page featuring someone from the firm who I thought was fairly good-looking: brown hair, strong arms crossed over the typical green plastic apron indicating mortuary work specifically. On closer inspection I read that this was Thomas, the embalmer of the company. Wanting to carry on the conversation I exclaimed 'Wow, who's the hottie?', at the same time as holding up the magazine for the rest of the girls to see – several of them, including the mortuary manager Tina, all sitting on chairs around the small office.

'That "hottie" is Tina's husband,' said Sharon, with a smile.

'Haha, come off it,' I scoffed, with a raised eyebrow. I really thought they were having me on, messing with the new girl.

'No, seriously,' Tina said, without a trace of a smile. 'That's my husband.'

I'd just called my new manager's husband a 'hottie'.
Great start to my first day.

When I say St Martin's was busy, that really is an understate-
ment. It was the mortuary of one of the largest hospitals in
London, but it also accepted Coronial cases from the local
jurisdiction, meaning some deceased came down from the
wards and some from the outside. Also, because it was an
established 'centre of excellence' when it came to High Risk
work – one of the main things I'd be doing as a Senior APT –
it also accepted deceased individuals from places as far away
as Brighton and Ipswich. I was never not busy. Our hours
were officially eight a.m. to four p.m. (unless we were on call)
but I'd religiously be in at seven thirty to make a pot of coffee
because, believe me, we were all going to need it. There were
many nights when I left nowhere near four but closer to six
or seven.

My usual routine was to carry out one or two High Risk
cases in the morning – tuberculosis, HIV and hepatitis
when I first started, as they were the most common daily
occurrence. I enjoyed the challenge immensely. High Risk
patients require their own room and equipment; they can't
be mixed in with other cases in the main post-mortem room
which trainee and Certificate holders are working in. The
St Martin's main autopsy suite was as large as the one at the
Metropolitan; larger, in fact, as it had a perinatal bench and
X-ray machine at the back (rather than in a separate room) as
well as a gallery for medical students to view post-mortems
as part of their training. But I loved having what felt like my
own personal autopsy suite – the High Risk room – to set
up for cases exactly as I wanted, while awaiting the arrival

of the hilarious, talented and enigmatic Professor Aloysius St Clare to carry out the examination. He wore a hat like Indiana Jones and sometimes, of all his garments, he'd take it off last in the High Risk changing room as he swapped his street clothes for scrubs. One day I walked in to find him in nothing but his boxer shorts and Indiana Jones hat, though he wasn't at all embarrassed. Hands on hips, he simply said, 'Carla, I think we'll need a lot of labels for this one. Lots of samples to take,' and I just looked all around the locker room at everything but his bare chest and pants and said shyly, 'Yes, Prof,' before dashing out of the room as quick as I could to print off labels, thankful for the excuse.

One of my new roles as Senior APT in this mortuary was to bury dead babies.

This was something I hadn't been expecting.

Every hospital has a Bereavement Centre, just like they'd had at the Metropolitan, but what I hadn't known was how closely this one and the mortuary department worked. For example, if the Bereavement Centre was completely over-whelmed and had lots of paperwork and we were quiet (not like *that* happened often), one of us would be expected to go upstairs and help them out. It was beneficial to us because we saw every single aspect of a patient's death and learned about all the relevant death administration.

Many hospitals have a fund they use to pay for very basic funerals for the deceased of their jurisdiction who are unclaimed. Or it may be that family members simply can't afford to do it themselves and meet government criteria for financial aid. The adult funerals were handled upstairs. What I had to do, sadly, was exactly the same thing for deceased babies but down in the mortuary, in the basement. I did not think there would be many situations in which parents wouldn't want to organise and directly oversee the funerals of their progeny – anything over twenty-four weeks' gestation came under my care, and anything under twenty-four weeks was under the care of Sharon – but it was a common occurrence and had me dealing with ten to fifteen perinatal funerals a month. I hadn't expected it because many funeral homes waive certain fees for baby and child burials, making them less expensive than the average ceremony – but still there were situations where I had to step in.

Organising these funerals usually involved lots of paperwork – everything in mortuary work does; it's the side that's never discussed – as well as a lot of contact with Anderson Morgan, who had the borough contract to carry out these ceremonies. I'd receive funeral request forms from the bereavement office via the maternity wards, then go and check the fridge to assess the size of the baby. As they'd be transported to Anderson Morgan via one of the temporary cardboard coffins, I'd then need to choose one for each tiny body, and that was always odd. Very small baby, eighteen or nineteen weeks? Definitely around a size 4 'shoebox'. Newborn, full term? More like a size 13. The bigger the baby, the bigger the cardboard box, and the harder it was for me to understand why the parents had seemingly abandoned their deceased child. I was, however, given all their details and I sent them letters via post and email instructing them of the time and place of the ceremony in case they wanted to come.

These tiny cadavers, which I came to call 'my babies', were collected monthly by a member of Anderson Morgan and I'd make sure I personally oversaw the process – the last part of my involvement with these apparently unwanted angels. I'd check every cardboard box and every ID band, tick each name off the list, then hand the whole batch over to the undertaker to be placed on an adult stretcher and covered with an elasticated topper. Then I'd mentally say my goodbyes.

When funeral directors came to collect the adult deceased, the procedure was similar: we'd answer the door, make chit-chat while we ensured the undertakers had the correct paperwork to state they could claim the deceased, and help them transfer the relevant patient over to their stretcher to be covered again by the topper. Various signatures were exchanged, a name – written in whiteboard marker – was rubbed off the fridge door, and the undertakers went on their merry way. It was sometimes difficult to remain friendly with all of them, especially the ones who seemed desperate to chat, when you were actually in the middle of an autopsy and you'd had to remove all your PPE to come out and deal with the situation – something I hadn't had to do at the Metropolitan. It's not malicious, it's just that your head is on your latest case and nothing distracts from it.

That's why I was surprised when Tina, who'd easily forgiven me for my initial faux pas about her 'hot' husband, came up to me one day with a playful glimmer in her eye.

'You know Sebastian?'

'No,' I said. I really didn't.

'You do,' she insisted. 'You were talking to him for ages yesterday. The southern one.'

'Tina, they're all really southern to me. I'm gonna need more.'

'Last Wednesday, you must remember.'

I thought for a moment, 'Ohhhh, yeah, I know. What about him?'

'Well he's asked Thomas to ask me if I can give him your phone number. He wants to ask you out.'

I tried to remember mine and Sebastian's various conversations over the last few months. Yeah, he was quite funny; there had been a bit of chemistry there, I thought. I remember he smelled nice. (Always good to be able to smell someone other than the deceased you're releasing.) It might seem weird to have flirty banter over cadavers in a hospital mortuary but no disrespect is meant by it. Love and death are intertwined in ways we can't even imagine. It's just the norm in that situation, the cycle of life in action. Plus it takes your mind off life's various atrocities. But did I want to go out with him if he couldn't even pluck up the courage to ask me out himself? Still, it was sweet . . .

My mind wandered back to the day I first saw Tina's husband Thomas in *Maxim*. She the mortuary manager, he the embalmer at the undertakers: it seemed like a match made in formaldehyde-scented heaven. When they were at home together they would be able to discuss everything that had happened at work and totally understand each other. It must be the best relationship in the world *ever*! I realised I wanted that. That's what had been lacking in my broken relationship and that's what I'd sought in my friendship with Josh. I wanted someone who could understand me and the job I loved, someone I could chat to properly about my working day. Sebastian was different from Thomas, who was quiet and shy; he was a bit of a lad, but he did make me laugh. Now that I'd remembered him I became quite keen on trying it out and seeing what it was like to be in that sort of relationship.

'OK, OK,' I said to Tina, who was looking at me with expectant glee. 'Fine – give him my phone number.'

So Sebastian and I dated; we were 'together'. I'd been in London for a while now and it was time for me to have a boy-friend. He lived with his parents and he drove so he usually came to see me or we'd meet up in central London. It was nice. We went out to eat and he always insisted on paying, we went shopping and he bought me gifts, he often turned up at my house with flowers, he took me to the cinema. We did all the things that young lovers do.

Sometimes, when I was in the PM room and the mortu-ary intercom buzzed, Sharon would shout, 'Lala, your other half is here!' (she always called me Lala rather than Carla), and I'd have the privilege of seeing my boyfriend at work. The novelty never wore off: I had another half! I was there-fore, by definition, whole. I loved my job, I liked my home, I had my own perfect formaldehyde-drenched relationship of mutual understanding like Tina and Thomas. I'd moved to London like Dick Whittington with nothing but the clothes on my back, a few books and some dreams – and I'd made it.

Life was good.

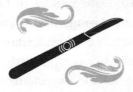

'Oh, for God's sake,' I moaned one morning, after opening up the fridge, 'the nurses have done it again.' I was looking at a deceased baby who'd been placed in the fridge overnight, wrapped in a blanket but with her tiny face left uncovered.

'What is it, Lala?' asked Sharon, walking over, measuring stick in hand. As soon as she saw the uncovered face of the baby she understood why I was annoyed.

The concept of 'dignity in death' is relative. Many of the nurses in hospitals I've worked in felt that babies shouldn't be placed in plastic body bags as it was 'too creepy', and many felt that their faces shouldn't be covered in the fridge at all as it was undignified: they wanted the babies on the trays to simply look like they were sleeping. The problem, which they weren't aware of because they weren't qualified APTs, is that the delicate facial skin of a baby can succumb to fridge burn, effectively disfiguring them and making it harder for the parents to view them. Despite the fact that we routinely gave new nursing staff official lectures on the topic during their induction, many still continued to leave babies' faces uncovered in the cold – a misplaced attempt at their idea of post-mortem decency.

'Well, at least this one isn't too bad,' Sharon continued. 'Not much damage.'

Still, it made me feel like all our efforts were being ignored. I covered the baby's face, sighed and slammed the fridge door shut, a little too hard. I think she could tell my mood wasn't really about the current issue, though, because she put the measuring stick down and asked, 'Lala – what's up?'

The truth was I hadn't been feeling myself for a while, and it wasn't being helped by Sebastian displaying some odd behaviour despite us having been together nearly ten months. Even though we spoke every day there had been a couple of times when he had completely disappeared for two or three days, falling off the face of the Earth. I'd had to have surgery on my birthday and had been unable to get hold of him that day or the next; no text or call from him asking if I was OK. He had disappeared again, which was making me understandably suspicious. Still, my mood really didn't seem like my own. I didn't like being made miserable and I had no idea what to do.

The decision was made for me anyway. That evening, I was caught completely unaware by a call to my mobile phone from an unknown number which I answered with the very customary 'hello'.

The return greeting was a rather uncustomary 'Are you Carla?' asked by a female in a spiteful tone. It caught me off guard. I skipped a beat before answering 'Yes', but I said it like a question, like I was unsure who I was when really I should have wondered who this curt person on my phone was.

'Can you tell me why my partner has your phone number written in a little black book which he hides under our bed? In our *home*? The place where our *child* sleeps?'

And I made a sound like a whimper as I dropped the phone.

The missing days.

The fact he always came to me.

The absence the night I'd had surgery.

It all began to make sense: I wasn't his girlfriend – I was the other woman.

Immediately after the phone call I felt odd. In fact, I'd never felt sicker in my life. It was as though the hands of some malignant entity had thrust rotten eggs, razor blades and maggots right through my abdominal skin into my stomach.

I felt the blood drain from my face – a cold, tingling sensation caused by that vital fluid leaving my capillaries and depriving my flesh of necessary oxygen. The blood also fled my extremities: icy pins and needles travelled from my fingers and toes, up my arms and legs until my abdomen was just one cold pit. I looked at my hands and my nails were blue. I was dazed. Where was my blood? Where could it possibly go? Was I going to vomit it out? No – the pressure in my chest made me feel like it was all in my heart; as if that resilient yet fragile organ Galen described was so stuffed with blood it couldn't beat and was close to bursting. But I also felt a heaviness in my lower belly that was so strong my hand groped beneath it protectively.

I stumbled into the bathroom and saw a corpse in the mirror, just like those I worked on daily: pale, waxy skin, sunken eyes, blue lips. I'd never fainted in my life but I'd seen other people do so and could partly understand what was happening. I slumped closer to the mirror. My pupils were so dilated my eyes had gone black. I stared and did not see myself reflected back: I saw something other, some shade of a person trapped inside the glass like Bloody Mary. I placed my hand on the mirror to steady myself, seeing at first only the beads of cold sweat on my upper lip; then, as I began to fall, I saw a smear of blood on my reflection. That crimson smear, glowing like fire in front of my icy countenance, was the last thing I saw.

I collapsed.

I was having a miscarriage.

I don't know how long I lay on the floor in the bathroom, the cheap bath rug my only source of comfort as I drifted in and out of consciousness. I don't think my lack of consciousness was due to a serious loss of blood. I simply just didn't want to wake up.

Not yet.

As a lawyer, my housemate, Denise, worked much longer hours than I did and when she finally came home she entered the bathroom to find me lying, ironically, in foetal position on the rug.

'Oh my God, Carla, what's happened?'

'I've had a miscarriage,' I answered, quietly. 'I don't know how . . . I didn't even know . . .' My sentences were trailing off because I didn't have the energy to finish them.

'We need to get you to a hospital!' Denise shrieked, as she fell down to her knees beside me.

The hospital was ten minutes away – I knew that because I used to work there. I had autopsied babies there.

I knew I had to go.

I was off work for a few days and in the interim I was prescribed anti-depressants, painkillers and sleeping tablets as well as antibiotics. They all danced in my stomach like fire imps because I was supposed to take them with food but I didn't want to eat. I didn't want anything.

Upon waking in the late afternoons I'd lie on my bed with the curtains open. I liked to watch the sky through the window particularly as twilight descended: there was something comforting about everything I could see being veiled in a dusky blanket, becoming darker and darker until nothing existed, only the moon. I reverted to something I hadn't considered in a long time for any form of comfort: religion. Not in a particularly coherent way; I just liked the feel of the cold haematite beads of my favourite rosary pressed against my feverish forehead. I took another sleeping pill at dusk, and as I began to fall asleep my fingers loosened their grip on the now warm beads. The last thing I'd see before my eyes closed was the blood of my miscarriage, still staining the underside of my fingernails.

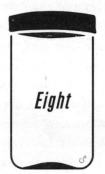

Eight

The Head: 'Losing My Head'

I don't wanna know your secrets,
They lie heavy on my head.

—Richard Ashcroft,
'Break the Night with Colour'

I was completely in the moment. The only thing I could do was focus; focus on the task at hand and take one minute at a time. I had already wet the hair of the deceased female lying on the tray and used a comb to create a horizontal parting at the back of her head – a thin thread of white skin connecting one ear to the other. With the same implement, I combed half of her hair forward over her face and half down the back of her neck, which was elevated up from the post-mortem table by a rubber head block. I swapped my comb for a scalpel, exactly traced the line of the parting with the blade, although with much more force, and the thin scalp yawned open, revealing the eggshell surface of the skull: a huge incision at the moment, but one that would be barely visible when reconstructed. Using one hand to grip the upper flap of scalp I pulled the skin over the top of the skull towards her face, with all my strength. There was a ripping sound and every now and again my progress would be foiled by some white connective tissues determined to keep the scalp attached to the bone. All it took to release them was a gentle caress of the blade, and the scalp would continue to peel forwards as I tugged hard, until the skull's bony forehead came into view. This was quite an easy head to open – I hadn't had to slice behind the ears for a bit of extra 'give'. Some heads are more difficult than others in that way. It made me think of a lovely APT from the Midlands who'd once joked to me, 'I think we should all be born with no ears and a zip.'

This was the way we dissected all adult heads. The large incision at the back could be stitched tidily after the examination and any hair combed down to cover it so it was hardly noticeable. If a decedent had very little or no hair we made the incision as far back as we could so that perhaps a pillow could hide it. We certainly never took the easy route and sliced through the forehead, something the creators of that movie prosthetic had wanted the world to believe ...

Using a similar technique, I also dissected the lower part of the incised scalp at the back of the head down towards the neck – a much easier task – then whipped my scalpel in a V-shape around the temporal muscles, both visible at the sides of the skull as two islands of striated muscle. These had to be dissected away from the bone and flattened against the displaced scalp to make way for what came next: the saw. Electric head saws used in autopsy rooms have oscillating blades, which means they can cut through bone but not skin or other soft tissue. They are, in fact, the same as those used to remove a plaster cast from someone's broken arm or leg after it has healed. Head saws create a lot of debris in the form of skull fragments and bone dust. For this reason, they often have a vacuum attachment and hooded suction tube to catch most of the dangerous particulate matter so that we APTs don't breathe it into our lungs, but it makes them incredibly loud and cumbersome. We can also opt to wear a paper surgical mask as well.

'Ready for me to remove the brain, Prof?' I asked, as I stood to attention, saw in hand like a member of the Queen's Guard holding a rifle. You always had to ask permission to begin this process because it also warned the doctor you were about to turn the saw on – very important given that he was handling sharp objects and the sudden electrical whining of a power tool could make him cut himself in fright if he wasn't expecting it.

'Yes, Carla, no problem,' Professor St Clare said.

He and I had a perfect rhythm going when it came to these High Risk cases in our small, specialised autopsy room, but we still ran through protocol. He'd barely finished his sentence before I turned the saw on. It whined like a dentist's drill yet growled like a vacuum cleaner. I manoeuvred the awkward hooded blade from the middle of the forehead in a straight line down to the left ear. I then did the same on the right. I repeated the process at the back of the skull: from the middle to the left ear and then to the right. This left me with an elliptical 'eye-shaped' piece of bone which was not quite free. There was one more thing to do: using the T-shaped

piece of metal, sometimes called a skull key, I inserted the
bottom of the letter T into the crevice created by the saw, hit
it with a mallet, and then, using the top of the T, I twisted to
the right. This immediately freed the skull from the tough
layer of tissue beneath it, called the dura, with a sound like a
crack and a rip at the same time. The skull cap – the calvarium – popped off easily and I laid it on the PM table beside
the deceased's head. I had revealed the glistening brain.

The brain looks so ... unassuming. It's hard to believe it
contains around a hundred billion neurons and is the source
of our personality, our memories – ourselves. Pink and shining, it seems almost a cheerful organ. Because it's so delicate,
I used one hand to hold it steady as I began to release it by
slicing through the cranial nerves at the centre of the base
of the skull. I then dug the scalpel deep into the foramen
magnum – the hole through which the brain joins the spinal
cord – and cut right across the cord to release it. I held it a
little to the left as I sliced through thin connective tissue
known as the tentorium on the lower right side of the skull,
and then repeated the process on the left. This then freed
the two cerebellar hemispheres making up the cerebellum,
the lower part of the brain, and I was able to place the whole
organ gently into the steel bowl of the weighing scales. Every
organ was weighed during the autopsy process and usually
the pathologist did that once he'd dissected them out of the
organ blocks. The brain was my job, though. I wrote '1349g'
on the whiteboard – an average weight for a brain, which is
usually between 1300g and 1500g – before carefully sliding
it on to the dissection board next to Prof and watching it
already begin to lose its shape; to deflate.

My brain felt like that: deflated and flat. But I don't think that was my real temperament – it was caused by the medication. Still, I was glad of the predictable daily insipidity. There were two things that could have made my return to work difficult. One was the ever-present threat that Sebastian might actually turn up. Everybody else in my mortuary seemed to be acting as though nothing had happened, as though I'd just been off with the flu, so why not him? The other was the fact that I had to continue my work burying babies. They were everywhere, these dead babies. I noticed them more now for obvious reasons: I had become a statistic. But I just felt numb thanks to the anti-depressants. I don't know what I would have felt had it not been for them. Every day I just wanted to come to work on time, do my job, and go home. I was like a zombie. I took my sleeping pill around six p.m. every evening, woke up the next day at five a.m., went to work and did the same zombie routine again. I was a very functional, hard-working zombie. I was a good zombie.

I suppose that's why I was fixated on the brain.

Prof snapped me out of it when he began slicing through the pink mass with a long, incredibly sharp brain knife, each thin segment of the organ flattening even further on to the bloody dissection board until it was just a pale puddle of mousse. He found nothing out of the ordinary. This was typical with High Risk cases such as this, which had been referred to us because of the patient's intravenous drug use, the inference being that if they've been using needles they could be HIV positive. The likelihood was that our patient had died of an overdose, but we could only say we suspected that cause of death 'pending toxicology'. I knew, therefore, what Prof was about to say before he said it, and I already had the syringe in my hand.

'Carla, we're going to need some vitreous,' he confirmed as he pulled off his latex gloves and threw them in the yellow clinical waste bin, then began furiously scribbling his findings on the autopsy form.

Although some APTs hated it, removing vitreous humor from the eyes was one of my favourite jobs because it required extra precision. Wielding my syringe, I moved around the steel post-mortem tray so I was face to face with my patient. When I looked into her crumpled visage it reminded me of my face: the stoic facade sometimes collapsing with tears once I got home at the end of the day when I really felt the loss of not one important thing in my life, but two.

I stopped thinking about that. Instead, I pulled her skin up and over the top of her open skull so she looked complete again and I could access her eyes. Then, after opening her eyelids wide with the fingers of one hand, with the other I took the needle and slid it sideways into the white of the eyeball – the sclera. The needle was horizontal and I could actually see it enter the eye via the clear lens; see it slide beneath the pupil. I then pulled on the syringe plunger to aspirate about two millilitres of the clear jelly known as vitreous humor, which is just one of the eye's components, along with aqueous humor, which has a more liquid consistency. Aqueous is replenished constantly but vitreous remains unchanged, so if there are drugs or other foreign bodies trapped in it they will stay there unless removed manually. That's why it's a valuable substance for toxicology testing. It also resists putrefaction longer than other body fluids and can even be examined after the deceased has been embalmed. I repeated the process with a different syringe on the other eye, and the samples of vitreous, along with others such as blood and urine, were ready to be sent to the toxicologist. Only then would we know if our patient was full of some unknown poison.

When I studied toxicology at university, I learned all about poisons. Absolutely anything can be a poison, even water; it all depends on what the dosage is. Paracelsus wrote about this in the sixteenth century and his words are often condensed into the Latin phrase *sola dosis facit venenum*, which means 'the dose makes the poison'. However, when we think of poisons and toxins we think of substances of abuse or classic stories of Agatha Christie-style villains administering strychnine, arsenic and cyanide. We think of inexorable, indiscriminate powders and liquids taking control of bodies and carrying out their dark deeds until the host is dead.

I was being poisoned.

Nearly every night I was receiving angry diatribes from Sebastian's common-law wife telling me secrets about him (via voicemail, since I never answered my phone), and although I didn't want to listen I couldn't help myself – it was a dark addiction. She was blurting out tales of how they'd been on family holidays, which explained those missing days, and the fact he'd taken her to see a show on my birthday – with tickets he said he'd bought for me. That was why he never contacted me about my surgery that day; once he realised I was in surgery he took her instead! She said how much he loved her because he had bought her a necklace from Tiffany's, but when she described it I knew it was the same one he'd bought me, too. It all just made me feel sick. Her words slid into my ear and entered my head like a black fungus, its mycelium hungry for more of my delicate pink brain matter, and once it had a grip I just didn't have the strength to fight it.

I did my work every morning on autopilot then on my lunch break, rather than eating, I drifted up to the hospital chapel like some pale spectre and lay on a pew for my designated hour. I went up there for the quiet; a sense of peace. I usually got it, but one day the Irish chaplain, Patrick, who I'd dealt with before for Catholic baby funerals, noticed that there was something very wrong with me as I lay horizontally, clutching my cold rosary against my forehead.

'Is everything OK?' he asked, softly. 'It's a stupid question, I know.'

I liked Patrick. He was a chaplain who wore a leather jacket and rode a motorcycle which made him cool in my books, as far as men of the cloth go.

I answered with a question: 'Have you ever felt that you've been close to someone who has done such filthy things that it's somehow rubbed off on you and become a part of you – that you can never be clean?'

I don't think he was prepared for that, but he said, after a pause, 'With God's help, you can always be cleansed. The mere fact of being in the presence of His grace can cleanse you.'

I thought about that for a moment but then, without saying a word, I put my rosary back in my scrubs pocket and headed back down to the mortuary.

It was that night I began compulsively bathing. I just didn't think I'd ever feel clean.

Pretty ironic, given that I'd spent all my adult life with the dead and knew about many cultures which have a 'taboo on the dead', whereby those who come into contact with the deceased are somehow 'unclean'. Sigmund Freud discussed this phenomenon, saying it exists because of 'the fear of the presence or of the return of the dead person's ghost', but this particular taboo has been around since long before Freud. In the Bible, the book of Numbers, chapter 19, verse 11 states 'The one who touches the corpse of any person shall be unclean for seven days', and verse 13 'Anyone who touches a corpse, the body of a man who has died, and does not purify himself, defiles the tabernacle of the Lord.' Haggai, chapter 2, verse 13, elaborates: "'If one who is unclean from a corpse touches any of these (bread, wine, oil) will the latter become unclean?" And the priests answered, "It will become unclean."'

And it's not just physical touching that causes problems: tribes such as the Tuareg in the Sahara fear the return of the dead so much they move their camp after a death and never speak the dead person's name. They wash the dead in the place they died, cover them in tree branches and the spot is considered a tomb for months. Similarly, there is a taboo on mourners and widows: the living should avoid them at all costs, lest they die themselves or suffer some awful fate. Even as recently as 2015, in Mumbai, around twenty-five Parsees, normally employed in jobs as varied as plumber and business-man, volunteered to work as khandias (pallbearers) because of an upcoming strike with the existing khandia workforce. An article commented, 'This is surprising considering the stigma attached to the profession – few Parsees are willing to marry khandias and orthodox members treat them as "untouchables".'

In an odd inversion to all these beliefs, the dead I was fine with – they'd never caused me any harm. It took a relation-ship with someone very much alive to make me feel tainted.

*

I felt like Tina was more understanding of my situation than the rest of the team and when she surprised me one day by asking, 'How do you fancy a day away from the mortuary to learn a new skill?' I replied, 'Sure,' thinking, '*Anything* to get out of here and away from everything, even for one day.'

'It's the enucleation course taught up in North London,' she continued. 'I know you like taking vitreous so I thought you could stomach this.'

Enucleation means removal of the eye and it's something that some mortuary technicians learn, even though there are designated eye-removal specialists at most tissue retrieval banks. Tina was right – I liked the accuracy and challenge of vitreous removal so eye retrieval was right up my street, and it's a real privilege to have a skill like that under your belt. It's carried out so that an organ donor can give the gift of their corneas to people who have conditions such as recurring infections and perforations which gradually cause a loss of vision.

So a few days later I was off to Hendon in North London. I used a fairly realistic plastic model called OSILA to practise removal techniques: the model face had fake optic nerves and various oblique and rectus muscles made of rubber and was as realistic as possible, even containing jelly-like slippery eyeballs and a conjunctiva. Like an 'alternative' Girl Guide, I coveted the certificate I received at the end of the day which told me I'd 'passed'. What a great skill to have and to put on my CV – and to bring up inappropriately at dinner parties! If only there was such a thing as an APT sash and we all earned patches for our achievements! I would have just earned the 'eye patch'.

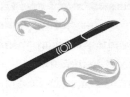

One very interesting post-mortem artefact of the eye is something known as *tache noire de la sclérotique*, meaning 'black spots of the eye' and often referred to as 'tache noire' for short. This occurs when the deceased's eyes are left slightly open and the sclera (the white part) becomes partially discoloured as it oxidises and dries out, usually around seven to eight hours after death. Rather than black spots, though, the exposed part of the eye becomes a red-brown line, as the delicate tissue succumbs to what's known as exposure keratitis. Because it looks like a rust-coloured straight line it's important to understand this phenomenon as a trained professional or it could easily be mistaken for some sort of injury or haemorrhage. A corneal transplant is usually rendered impossible by this damage unless the keratitis affects just the sclera and not the cornea; in that case it may be possible. So that's one of the reasons it's important to close the eyes of the deceased. Although it's said that as a matter of tradition coins were placed on the eyes of the dead to stop them reflecting on the living and passing on the condition, as well as to pay the Ferryman in Hades, it's also just highly practical.

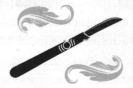

I tried to keep the personal problems I was having away from the workplace and continued to run around the mortuary at St Martin's like a headless chicken. Keeping busy seemed to be the only thing keeping me sane.

There's a famous case of a headless chicken that lived for well over a year. In 1945, in Colorado, farmer Lloyd Olsen was assigned the task by his wife of killing one of the brood for supper, but he didn't quite chop the head off properly and left some of the jugular vein as well as most of the bird's brain stem intact. Because of this the chicken, who was called Mike, was able to walk clumsily, balance on a perch and even attempt to crow, although the noise apparently came out as a hideous gurgling sound. Olsen decided to feed Mike with tiny grains of corn, as well as a mixture of milk and water via an eyedropper, to keep him alive. He exhibited him in carnivals for the eighteen months that Mike 'lived' and made himself a lot of money, but the creature unfortunately (or fortunately, depending on how you view such a horrible existence) died one night after choking on a kernel of corn.

I'm often asked if I've ever autopsied someone who has been beheaded, and if the process works the other way round. Of course, humans cannot live without a head, but there remains a curiosity as to whether or not the head, once decapitated, is still sentient – at least for a short while.

In Paris, in April 1792, the infamous guillotine was used for the first human execution after a couple of weeks of trials on animals and corpses. It was named after Dr Joseph-Ignace Guillotin, who did not actually invent the instrument – many other beheading apparatuses had existed for years, including the Italian 'Mannaia' (cleaver), the Scottish 'Maiden' and the Halifax 'Gibbet' – but Guillotin supported its use as he believed decapitation was a much more humane way to bring about instantaneous death. It therefore became the preferred form of capital punishment. Hanging, used in pre-revolutionary France, on the other hand, was fraught with problems. There were several different methods of judicial hanging but the 'Long Drop' or 'Measured Drop' became the standard method in the UK as it was considered the most humane. Unlike earlier methods, this one took the person's height and weight into consideration. It meant that the rope was the right length to ensure a correct and speedy hanging, but it didn't result in the decapitation of the victim which, ironically, occurred frequently, even in France. So the guillotine was perceived to be more merciful as it delivered an immediate death without risk of suffocation.

However, three years after the guillotine's debut a letter, written by the eminent German anatomist Samuel Thomas von Sömmerring, was published in the *Paris Moniteur*, which stated:

> Do you know that it is not at all certain when a head is severed from the body by the guillotine that the feelings, personality and ego are instantaneously abolished ... ? Don't you know that the seat of the feelings and appreciation is in the brain, that this seat of consciousness can continue to operate even when the circulation of the blood is cut off from the brain ... ? Thus, for as long as the brain retains its vital force the victim is aware of his existence ... Credible witnesses have assured me that they have seen the teeth grind after the head has been separated from the trunk.

The medical community was in a panic as stories of this disturbing phenomenon spread like wildfire. After Charlotte

Corday was guillotined for murdering the revolutionary Jean-Paul Marat in his bath, the executioner slapped her cheek while holding her severed head aloft. Witnesses claimed 'the cheeks reddened and the face looked indignant'. (I think I would too if I'd just been executed and the cherry on top of the cake was a slap.) According to another tale, when the heads of two rivals in the National Assembly were placed in a sack following execution, one bit the other so badly the two couldn't be separated.

While it is true that the brain can stay oxygenated by the blood within it for up to twelve seconds after decapitation, it isn't quite so cut and dried as to whether that brain retains conscious thoughts. Gruesome experiments were carried out on animals and criminals in an attempt to answer the question once and for all, but no real evidence emerged that one decapitated head could indeed bite another. Scientists now believe that the huge drop in cerebral blood pressure would cause a victim to lose consciousness in a few seconds, so hopefully a few seconds is quick enough . . .

I find it interesting that the innocent attraction, Madame Tussaud's Waxwork Museum, began due to these beheadings. In the 1790s a lack of media meant that most of the population didn't know what the aristocracy looked like, unlike today when their images are everywhere. So the talented Marie Tussaud, after escaping execution by guillotine herself owing to her artistic skills, was employed to collect the heads and make plaster casts of them which she subsequently used to make wax models. Eventually, after escaping France, she took them on a travelling exhibition and finally settled at her famous Marylebone Road location.

*

Not only casts and waxworks, but heads themselves, have been a commodity throughout history. Examples include *kapala*, ritual skull cups made from ornately decorated human calvaria and used commonly in Tibet, and the mainly Amazonian practice of shrunken heads. One particularly contentious form of head trading occurred in New Zealand in the early 1800s, around the time of the European invasion. At this time some Maori tribe members – women and men – had their faces tattooed and incised with what is known as moko. These distinct markings identified the tribe members, particularly if their heads had been severed, and the preservation of these heads after death became an important part of Maori post-mortem culture. After the brain and eyes had been removed and the orifices sealed, the heads were boiled or steamed, then smoked over a fire and left out to dry in the sun. The result was a mummified head with the moko beautifully preserved. These *mokomokai* would be brought out of safekeeping for important occasions, and the invading Europeans began to trade their muskets for them. Before long, owing to their intricate beauty, they were a desired commodity for people travelling from the West. When the supply of genuine heads diminished as a result, *mokomokai* had to be 'created'. Unfortunately, for many slaves this was the only way in which they would receive the moko: they were tattooed, allowed to heal, then promptly beheaded and their heads treated in the way described above to be sold on as chiefs to unsuspecting collectors.

An amusing exchange is documented by Frederick Maning in his book *Old New Zealand*. He thought he had stumbled into a circle of Maori who were nodding to him in greeting. It turned out to be *mokomokai* bobbing on fabric-swathed sticks in the gentle breeze. As this realisation hit him, he heard a voice from behind:

'Looking at the 'eds, sir?'

'Yes,' said I, turning round just the least thing quicker than ordinary.

''Eds has been a-getting scarce,' says he.

'I should think so,' says I.

'We an't 'ad a 'ed this long time,' says he.

'The devil!' says I.

'One o' them 'eds has been hurt bad,' says he.

'I should think all were, rather so,' says I.

'Oh no; only one of 'em,' says he. 'The skull is split, and it won't fetch nothin',' says he.

'Oh, murder! I see, now,' says I.

''Eds was werry scarce,' says he, shaking his own ''ed'.

'Ah,' said I.

'They had to tattoo a slave a bit ago,' says he, 'and the villain ran away, tattooin' an' all!' says he.

'What?' said I.

'Bolted afore he was fit to kill,' says he.

'Stole off with his own head?' says I.

'That's just it,' says he.

'Capital felony!' says I.

I walked away, pretty smartly. 'Loose notions about heads in this country,' said I to myself.

Although this is a comical dialogue, the traffic in these once-revered objects did become a public scandal, on a par with the modern Alder Hey scandal, when it became known that the practice had cost many innocent people their lives.

An act made their repellent trade illegal in 1831. Now, museums in England do what they can to repatriate these remains to their country of origin.

In Oscar Wilde's play *Salomé*, based on the short biblical tale from Mark 6:21–29, the arrogant and passionate princess Salomé demands the head of the prophet John the Baptist (Jokanaan) on a silver platter. She wants him beheaded because he will not kiss her: he is a holy man and sees her lust for him as something dirty and unholy, and he doesn't want her to taint him. The decapitation is her revenge. As she holds his severed head in front of her face, she declares, 'Ah! thou wouldst not suffer me to kiss thy mouth, Jokanaan. Well! I will kiss it now', and other sexually charged taunts which go on for many lyrical lines.

The reason I know this story is fictional is because Salome, back in the days when tricep dips and bicep curls were not common practice for young princesses, would not have had the upper-body strength to keep holding a human head in front of her face long enough to have a lengthy conversation with it.

And I know that because I've held a decapitated head in my hands.

Many years ago, when I was at the Municipal Mortuary, I spent some time over at the local hospital facility with Jason, in order to train for forensic post-mortems. They were held there because their mortuary was much bigger than ours and had specific equipment for these special cases, such as a viewing gallery from which police could watch autopsies without getting 'dirty', and CCTV for evidence purposes. When we arrived at about two in the afternoon I was surprised to see so many people there: the pathologist going over video footage and photographs of the crime scene with the senior investigating officer (SIO) and several other police colleagues, the photographer and assistant setting up their equipment, and all the exhibits officers and note-takers preparing for the arduous examination. Once the body bag was opened – this has to be done on film, with witnesses, to establish chain of evidence – I was even more surprised to see that the deceased had no head. Scratch that: on further inspection he *did* have a head, but as it was separate from his body it had been placed between his legs in an attempt to stop it rolling around in the bag. It seemed completely logical, although it was an odd experience to have someone staring at me from below their own genitals. The urge to pick it up and move it into the correct anatomical position was strong but I wasn't able to touch anything yet – not until everyone was ready to begin the autopsy.

In forensic cases, after the pathologist has carried out the external exam, it is he who also carries out the evisceration. Everything on or in the deceased needs to be noted by a medical doctor qualified in Forensic Pathology as they may need to testify in court. It's not a responsibility APTs are trained for. One thing we still do, however, is dissect the head to remove the brain, but in this case I assumed it wouldn't be requested. The man had been murdered – someone had chopped his head off with a very sharp blade – and it was now up to the police to discover who did it. When they eventually did, the pathologist would be called to present his findings to a jury in court.

Case closed, hopefully.

Imagine my surprise when Dr Colin Jameson said, 'OK guys, you can crack on with the head.'

I looked at Jason, eyes wide with fear, thinking, 'How the hell are we going to do that here?' As if Jason could read my mind, he said calmly, 'Right, you get the saw and I'll hold him.'

I moved closer to Jason and whispered that I didn't feel comfortable wielding the cumbersome saw in front of all these people – I was still a trainee at the time and I was used to my heads being attached to something.

'OK, you hold him and I'll saw,' he said. 'But you really need to hold on tight.'

So I found myself across the post-mortem table from Jason, holding a heavy, decapitated head aloft, manoeuvring it into the right position then keeping it steady on the stainless steel. I needed to be careful that my fingers didn't stray past the deceased's ears because I would have lost them to Jason's scalpel so, weirdly, I had to hold this decapitated head like I would a lover: by placing both hands on his cheeks. I then had to lean forward and rest my elbows on the steel in order to balance myself and strengthen my grip. I was staring directly into the eyes of this severed head as though I was about to kiss him, just like Salomé, and there were around twelve pairs of eyes on me as I carried out this odd and intimate task. As if that wasn't bad enough, my bottom was in the air. It would have been like a comedy sketch if the circumstances hadn't been so harrowing.

Jason was right. As he made the incision and reflected the scalp I found I was capable of holding the head steady, but as soon as he started to saw I just didn't have the strength to compete with it. The sheer force of the machinery kept making me tilt the head so Jason couldn't create a straight line. So we had to swap, and I sawed through the skull while he held the man's head with his body-builder's hands and forearms. Eventually we had the calvarium off and the brain in the scales and, sweating and red-faced, I felt like I'd passed some sort of test. Reconstruction was going to be interesting ...

One other thing that was odd (as if the whole situation wasn't bizarre enough) was the removal of the neck and tongue organs, or what we call the pharynx – the throat. There are a couple of ways to do this. When I did a typical Y-incision on a decedent propped up on a rubber block, it created a triangular flap of skin over the whole neck, the 'point' of which was near the middle of the clavicles. You can feel the place yourself as the dip between your own collarbones – it's called the suprasternal notch. I'd take the tip of this skin triangle between my fingers or toothed forceps and pull upwards towards the face, all the while freeing the white connective tissue clinging to the sternocleidomastoid (SCM) muscles of the neck in the same way the scalp clung to the skull. It took just a feather-light touch of a sharp scalpel to help me progress. I'd continue this way until the jawbone of the deceased was visible like a large white wishbone, and the neck muscles completely uncovered. Then, taking a PM40, I'd slide the blade under the jawbone (into the mouth – I could see the shining blade skimming behind the teeth) and cut along it from one end to the other, allowing me to pull the tongue down and under the mandible. I'd then slice across the back of the mouth and pull all the neck structures away from the bone – tongue, larynx, trachea, SCMs – just working my way down and eventually revealing the vertebrae behind the tissues.

However, a straight or I-incision stops at the suprasternal

notch so this process is infinitely more difficult. Effectively I'd have to carry out the whole process blind. Because I couldn't cut the skin of the neck I had to force the PM40 beneath the neck skin, find the jawbone with the blade and cut along it without seeing what I was cutting, using the bone as a guide. All the while I'd have to make sure I didn't perforate the neck skin, therefore making the whole point of the straight incision useless. (Although that superglue I mentioned was definitely a lifesaver when it came to nicks like that, which we called 'buttonholes' – it could make an incision practically invisible or simply look like a natural wrinkle.)

But what were we to do in this situation? The poor man's tongue and half his pharynx were in the head and the rest of it was in the body.

I just said to Jason, 'Bagsy the body,' since that was completely opened. I'd let him struggle with trying to remove half a pharynx from a decapitated head in front of all these glaring eyes.

We remove the neck and tongue routinely in autopsies for many reasons; nothing is done gratuitously. First we check in the mouth to see that there is no food or other foreign matter, which could indicate choking. But superficially looking into the mouth cavity is not enough. By removing the pharynx the pathologist can open it up to see if there's a bolus of food stuck in the oesophagus or the trachea. For example, some onlookers may witness what they think is the victim of a cardiac arrest but at autopsy we discover cause of death to be what's known as a café coronary. This occurs when an intoxicated person chokes on her food and the natural gag reflex is suppressed by the alcohol in the blood. (Now you see why food and death are so interconnected for me – there are just so many associations!) The tongue can also be checked for artefacts like bite marks: if a decedent bit their own tongue they may have had a seizure. The delicate cartilage and hyoid bone of the larynx may be damaged in the case of mechanical choking by another individual, and classically, the way to determine if a victim of a fire was alive during it is to find sooty deposits in the trachea which indicate breathing in smoke. There is so much to be discovered just in that one small part of the body which not many people realise we remove at autopsy.

Perhaps, then, one of the most important things when working in a mortuary is being able to 'keep your head', to focus in the face of some of the strangest or most gruelling deaths that can be experienced. It's bad enough reading about some cases in the paper; imagine what it's like for the families of the victims and for those in the death industry who see everything right there in front of them. Up until the later part of my career I felt like I'd been keeping a fairly good balance, teetering on the edge of the two abysses: one, caring too much and having a nervous breakdown, and the other, caring too little and becoming callous and detached. But recent events in my life had started to make me rethink my job. I no longer felt balanced enough to deal with the stresses coming my way. I was, in effect, starting to lose my own head.

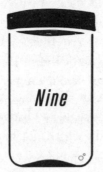

Nine

Fragmented Remains: 'Bitsa'

Bitsa this, bitsa that. Put 'em all together and
what've you got?

—*Bitsa (kids' TV show theme)*

In southern Africa there is a form of traditional medicine
which sometimes rears its ugly head among the populace.
It's a type of witchcraft containing rogue aspects as well as
the traditional medicine magic, 'Muti', said to be extremely
potent because it requires body parts of the dead. The only
time Muti becomes familiar to the mainstream in the developed world is when a ritualistic 'medicine murder' hits the
headlines. Take, for example, the heinous case in 2001 of
the 'Torso in the Thames', in which a small, headless and
practically limbless torso was discovered in London's famous

river, still wearing a pair of orange shorts over the stumps of his legs. Realising it was the body of a child and unwilling to allow him to disappear into obscurity, investigators decided to name him Adam. It required scores of experts deploying a multitude of analytical and investigative techniques to uncover some truths about the unidentified remains. A sophisticated analysis of Adam's bones for trace minerals absorbed from nutrition revealed levels of strontium, copper and lead two and a half times higher than would normally be expected in a child living in England. From that analysis, forensic geologists gradually narrowed down Adam's likely origin to West Africa, probably Nigeria. Then forensic work carried out by botanists at Kew Gardens identified unusual plant extracts found in Adam's intestine as those which grow only in the area around Benin City, the capital of Edo State in southern Nigeria. It took many years, but Adam was eventually tentatively identified as Patrick Erhabor, and he was no longer just a torso. It was claimed he was a young boy who had been trafficked to the UK from Nigeria specifically for a ritual sacrifice.

The case lifted the lid on abhorrent Muti practices, such as the kidnapping and murder of a ten-year-old South African girl, Masego Kgomo, in 2009, which happened in order to sell some of her body parts to a sangoma, a practitioner of the tradition. This case sparked calls to sangomas to stop the practice.

Only two years ago I nearly spat out my coffee while checking my morning news alerts before heading into work: the headline screamed 'Genitals Stolen from Morgue!' Upon reading it, I discovered that the breasts and labia had been removed from the dead bodies of two elderly women in

Durban, South Africa, and the writer speculated that the crime was Muti-related. According to another article, 'it is often soft tissues such as eyelids, lips, scrota and labia which are excised from the dead for these practices' – practices which clearly still continue.

When I first began working in mortuaries I was usually confronted with the totality of death – and the deceased – as a whole. It isn't commonplace in the UK to experience cases which involve fragmented remains, although in other parts of the world the likelihood may be higher. Therefore, I never really considered people in pieces – not until the morning I opened the furthest door of the fridge unit at St Martin's and discovered a large, bright-yellow plastic tub. It was about two feet high by three feet wide.

'This is a pretty big sharps bin!' I shouted to Sharon. 'What's it doing in the fridge?'

A sharps bin is a bright-yellow plastic container used specifically for the disposal of scalpel and PM40 blades, as well as needles from syringes and even broken glass. It basically does what it says on the tub, in big black letters. But I realised this huge version didn't have 'Sharps Bin' written on it, at about the same time as Sharon walked over to see what I was referring to.

Her throaty laugh echoed around the fridge room before she answered in her comforting cockney accent, 'What are you like, Lala? That ain't a sharps bin!'

'Well, what is it?'

'It's a limb bin.'

Situations like this are one of the reasons I love working in different mortuaries. No matter how much you think you know, there's always something else to learn. A limb bin, I discovered, is a temporary storage unit for parts of bodies that have been surgically amputated – meaning they're usually found in hospitals. Amputation occurs more frequently than you might assume: for example, after an accident if a person's hand or arm has been damaged beyond repair, or, in the case of diabetes, when peripheral arterial disease (PAD) causes blood loss to the foot and lower leg, and ultimately ulcers and necrosis.* Although the patients usually haven't died from the procedure there's nothing that can be done with the appendages, so they're brought down to the mortuary on adult stretchers covered in a white sheet. They are then unveiled by the porter assigned this odd task, with an ostentatious flourish, as though he's in a posh hotel delivering room service to Hannibal Lecter.

'Can I see inside?' I asked. I imagined the contents to be something Dr Frankenstein would keep in his turret-based laboratory, picturing in my head a mish-mash of arms and legs crossed over each other, hands intertwined around feet, and maybe the odd finger or toe. In my head I heard John Goodman in *The Big Lebowski* saying, 'You want a toe? I can get you a toe.'

'Course you can,' said Sharon as she removed the lid.

I peered over the top, like a child would with a toy box, but I was slightly disappointed. Of course, the limbs weren't just flailing about like some nightmarish vision from a Marquis de Sade novel; they were all wrapped up and neatly packaged, looking more like parcels in a mail room. I learned from

---

* The charity Diabetes UK recently released information stating that diabetes-related amputations had reached an all-time high of 135 a week.

Sharon that once the bin is full, all these extraneous body parts are sent to be incinerated in the bowels of the hospital. At the time I thought, 'What a waste.' I don't know what I was envisaging could be done with these leftover limbs, because creating a monster à la Dr Frankenstein was obviously out of the question – not enough thunder and lightning in the UK, for a start – and I supposed they weren't suitable for trainee doctors to practise dissection on because they had far too many disfiguring injuries. It's only very recently, 2016 in fact, that a genius use for these wasted limbs was proposed.

In the UK we do not have forensic taphonomy facilities, colloquially known as 'Body Farms' (the first and most famous one was created by forensic anthropologist Dr Bill Bass in Tennessee). These facilities are vital for gathering data on the various ways a cadaver can decay, and this data can be used to try to pinpoint time of death and therefore possibly establish or destroy the alibis of perpetrators of crimes. At the moment our laws in the UK do not permit such a facility, and instead we use pigs.

But humans aren't pigs. OK, *some* are, but not physiologically. Recent studies at that Tennessee facility compared pig to human decomposition and the rates are not the same – in fact they vary wildly. This has serious negative implications for the use of pig data in courts worldwide. Quite simply, we can't keep using pigs as human analogues for forensic taphonomy research – that is, the study of burial, decay and preservation. So a leading forensic anthropologist, Dr Anna Williams, and her student, cadaver dog expert Dr Lorna Irish, proposed a fantastic idea: what about populating a 'Body Farm' with human limbs and tissue removed surgically, instead of allowing them to be incinerated in our limb bins? Their decay rates could be studied and cadaver and victim recovery dogs could be trained on the real thing.

I undergo facial surgery quite frequently. I suffer with a rare but non-life-threatening neurocutaneous disorder called Parry-Romberg Syndrome which means I've had pieces of muscle fascia (a collagen-rich connective tissue which surrounds the muscles) removed from both my thighs and temporal muscles and implanted into atrophying parts of my face. It wouldn't have bothered me if any of my surplus tissue from these procedures had been used for research in the above way rather than simply being incinerated; indeed, I'd have liked an option to say so. I may well be a scientist fighting on the side of forensics progress, but I'm also a patient. I'm human, made of flesh and bone, and helping other humans is a priority.

An article about this proposal stated, 'This new suggestion of allowing volunteers to donate body parts following operations is being seen as a "halfway house approach", which scientists claim could prove invaluable in advancing forensic work.' It would be one step closer to using whole donors and one step closer to smashing the taboo of using the dead for research. A survey carried out within the article showed that 94 per cent of respondents considered it a good idea, agreeing with the comment 'If they're going spare, why not?' Only 6 per cent found the idea 'gruesome and creepy'. Perhaps the notion that these human remains aren't from deceased individuals removes some of the stigma, especially that left by the organ retention scandal and Alder Hey, and makes it easier to swallow?

Actually, 'easier to swallow' is a poor turn of phrase to use when talking about amputated extremities. At the Pathology

Museum, when I teach the history of 'potting' human specimens from the 1600s onwards, I discuss the first preservative
used for teaching – alcohol, also known as 'spirits of wine' –
and bring the process right up to date with an imaginary
trip to the Yukon, in Canada. In Dawson City there is a bar
called the Eldorado. In this bar, a drink of any choice of alcohol containing a real severed human toe is served to patrons
who want to take part in the Sourtoe Challenge. The rules
are, 'You can drink it fast, you can drink it slow, but your lips
have gotta touch the toe!'

The story began in the 1920s when rum-runner and
miner Louis Liken had his frost-bitten toe amputated and he
decided to keep it as a souvenir in alcohol, as you do. Many
years later, in 1973, Yukon local Dick Stevenson found the
toe and thought, 'Hey, why not put it in a drink and create a
challenge?' Again – as you do. Thus the Sourtoe Cocktail was
born, and to this day those who manage the feat of drinking
one are presented with a certificate stating that they belong to
the Sourtoe Cocktail Club. However, disaster struck in 1980
when a challenger's chair tipped back as he was drinking and
he swallowed the toe. Records state that 'Toe Number One
was never recovered'!

Helpfully, the living flooded the bar with toe donations
(toe-nations?). One was amputated due to diabetes, one
due to an inoperable corn (urgh), and one simply arrived
anonymously in a jar of alcohol with a note giving the sage
advice: 'Don't wear open-toe sandals while mowing the lawn'.
Recently, though, the ninth toe was swallowed – seemingly
on purpose, for the swallower had to pay a $500 fine. That
fine has since been increased to $2500 to ensure their back-up
tenth toe doesn't disappear along with all the others.

Anyway, the point is that instead of just incinerating live patients' parts – or using them for drinking games – let's put them to good, forensic use.

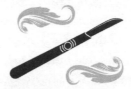

People sometimes come into the mortuary fragmented due to a horrible occurrence like an accident or a suicide, the most frequent being RTIs (road traffic incidents), railway incidents or 'jumpers'.

One suicide I remember in particular was a man who had thrown himself in front of an oncoming tube train, which in London is euphemistically known as 'a person under a train'. When this occurs, passengers on the platform tend to be informed via loudspeaker, 'The service has severe delays due to a person under a train', as though they're just hiding under there for a bit, or perhaps having a picnic. Death is still so taboo that Transport for London won't simply say 'due to a death'.

On opening the body bag at autopsy we were confronted with the extent of the suicide's fragmentation: the upper left of his skull was destroyed, both hands were hanging off his wrists, attached by a few tendons and some skin, and his body was split across his middle which had caused his behind to spin around to his front; that is, my eyes travelled from his crushed head, down his mangled torso and straight to his buttocks. His genitals were somewhere at the back, underneath him (I hoped, for his sake). He also had one foot completely severed at the ankle and one lower leg off at the knee, both placed in correct anatomical position in the body bag. I think. It was hard to tell because his legs were the wrong way round. To top it off, we could see through the mangled chest and abdominal cavity that most of his organs were missing. However, there were several plastic evidence bags within the body bag containing, as far as we could ascertain, his organs and other fleshy debris which the British Transport Police (BTP) and the recovery team had scraped up from the surrounding area.

All in all, it was a mess. But we still had to carry out a post-mortem.

First, we had to determine exactly which organs were missing. Some, like the two kidneys, were still intact inside his body cavity. Because they're positioned at the back (retro-peritoneal area) of the body and surrounded by a thick layer of fat they are quite protected compared to other organs. In this case they had clung to his back, like two limpets. The spleen, on the other hand, was gone. It's such a delicate organ that it can be one of the first to be injured or completely obliterated – many people will have heard the term 'ruptured spleen'. I imagined his was squished somewhere along the train track, leaving a sad, dark red smear.

I sighed as I sifted through the small bags and found some remnants of his brain, his heart, and other pieces of tissue that I couldn't differentiate from one another.

'Prof, I think you're going to need to look through these bags,' I said, frustrated by what seemed like an impossible jigsaw. I took my gloves off so I could wipe my brow. 'Your eye is better than mine at working out what some of these pieces are anyway.' In truth, I could probably have done it, but it was bringing back some bad memories.

People in pieces. It was nothing new to me.

When I'd worked in the temporary mortuary after the 7/7 bombings we sadly dealt mainly with fragments of human beings, especially towards the end: small plastic bags of unidentified material scraped from the four different detonation sites. Combined with what the recovery teams had assumed were the remains of victims were bones from wild creatures that had died in the tunnels (rats, pigeons, mice), bones and meat from discarded Kentucky Fried Chicken meals or similar, and other objects that were not even animal but vegetable or mineral. Add to that the fact that those responsible also blew themselves up and there was the very real possibility their remains had commingled with those of their victims.

Such a horrible way to go: to not only be blasted into pieces but to be mixed in with everyday detritus, even pieces of your murderer.

What a terrible crime.

We did everything humanly and mechanically possible. We sifted through those bags, we identified tissues and bones that were human, and we passed them on to the anthropologists and other specialists further down the facility if we weren't sure. We tagged everything separately, we sent them for DNA testing, and the results were compared with members of families that had either confirmed they'd lost someone to the blast or had someone still missing.

It's not easy to hear or discuss such details. I could, of course, go into much more detail, but I won't, for reasons I gave earlier in the book. Nonetheless, it's important people appreciate the lengths the professionals went to in order to reunite those fragmented remains with their source and ensure no one was laid to rest with a remnant that didn't belong to them. It's crucial to know the realities of these crimes, particularly terror attacks, which play, in part, on that age-old fear of being fragmented in death, or of perhaps leaving no remains and therefore nowhere for next of kin to mourn.

I put on a fresh set of gloves now that I'd had a moment to stretch my hands and breathe, and turned my attention back to Railway Man. It was fairly evident the cause of death, according to the pathologist, was 'extensive and severe blunt force trauma', and the manner of death was Suicide (as opposed to Accident, Natural Causes, Homicide or Unascertained). In the UK, the manner of death has usually been identified at this point by a legal officer, such as the Coroner.

Professor St Clare had thankfully told me there was no need to 'open' the head since we could see inside anyway and his brain was already 'removed'. That was beneficial for my reconstitution of the deceased later. It didn't take Prof long to fill out the form and take it with him as he removed his PPE and headed up to his office to write his report. I was left alone not only with Railway Man, but a dissection bench, cutting board, sink, walls and equipment all covered in blood and pieces of tissue. My priority was to ensure the blood didn't dry on the various surfaces and stick to them so first I gathered together every single piece of excess flesh and placed them in a steel bowl with the rest of my patient's organs. I even used forceps to pick up the smallest remnants I could find. They would all be dealt with during the reconstruction. In autopsy rooms we use hoses attached to the dissecting benches to clean down. They usually have spray nozzles with trigger handles to control the flow of the water. I picked up the hose and began to spray all the surfaces down thinking, with typical dark humour, that it was a metaphor for my life right then: me being left alone to clean up a mess somebody else had made.

I knew at some point I had to take some responsibility for the mess that had been my relationship and the effect it had had on me. The thoughts going round my head about it somehow being my fault, and how I should have been more vigilant, and how on earth I could have been the last to know about the situation, were ruining my days – but what was worse was that I was letting them. I decided that, rather than try to desensitise myself and prolong the process of 'grief', or whatever it was I was feeling, I'd just come off the meds, do some cold turkey, and get through it on my own. I kept thinking of that Winston Churchill quote: 'If you're going through Hell, keep going.' I figured things couldn't get worse, so that was that. 'Adios, Prozac. Time to move on.'

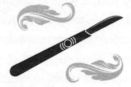

I opened the fridge one morning to see for myself a mistake I had assumed had been made on my baby funeral paperwork. I was supposed to organise a funeral for a child aged two and a half years. That couldn't be right: surely they meant two and a half months? On unzipping the small white body bag I was shocked to see the most beautiful baby boy. His blond hair was curled against the marble of his forehead like one of Botticelli's angels, and the eyelashes of his closed eyes were so long they caressed his plump cheeks like tiny, dark kisses. I wanted to kiss those cheeks. I was overcome with sorrow for this cherubic child who had been abandoned in death for unknown reasons and left in my care – the care of a stranger – for 'disposal'. A sob escaped me, and it echoed around that cold fridge room, ricocheting off each white door so that by the time it reached my ears again it was unrecognisable.

'I don't cry,' I thought. 'I have a job to do.' But even as I heard the words in my head I was scooping the cold, dead toddler out of the fridge and my tears were falling, creating cerulean circles on his pale blue baby-gro.

I think I was crying for a hundred reasons. I was pressing his frigid body to me in a warm embrace and weeping because I wondered where his parents or other family were and why they weren't dealing with his funeral. I was crying for that 'fish-baby' I'd witnessed that perinatal pathologist throw on to the weighing scales like she was at a deli counter; crying for every single perinatal post-mortem I'd done in the last few years; and crying for the one baby I hadn't even been able to keep safe – my own.

When you work with the dead you cannot weep for every single case you encounter – you'd be utterly useless. It's a defence mechanism that works perfectly well until something just snaps and tells you, 'OK, it's time: now have a cry, then get back to it.'

This was one of those times, and I just came apart.

I cried for every deceased patient I'd ever worked on and every one of their family members or friends. I think I also cried for myself: for the long work days, coming in up to an hour early in the morning just so I could try to catch up on paperwork before the fax and the phone began ringing and the others turned up and the pandemonium started again. I cried because of the weekends when I felt lonely in a city I had yet to figure out. I cried because I felt unsupported by the girls I worked with. I cried because I'd come off the medication and was feeling the intensity of my emotions for the first time in a long time. I cried because – who knows? I just needed it.

I kept going until I had run out of tears, then I wiped my face with the sleeve of my white coat and placed the angelic baby back into the fridge with the teddy bear in his arms. I also covered his face and zipped up the body bag to make sure there would be no fridge burn on those perfect cheeks. It wasn't much; just one small gesture to encompass a world of grief. And then, like I always did – like we all always do – I moved on.

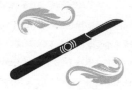

At this point I wasn't to know that things would get so much better; that I'd spend the next years of my career surrounded by fragmented human remains at the Pathology Museum, yet still feel completely whole. It hadn't even been in my 'career plan'. But something or someone had a plan for me and it exposed me to yet more death contemplation and research. There was so much more to learn from fragmented bodies that had withstood preservation for one to two hundred years, because the reasons for their procurement were so different from remains I'd dealt with at autopsy or helped remove for histological analysis. The preservation or 'potting' procedures used at Bart's were old and varied wildly, meaning I would be able to focus more on the history of dissection and display rather than current guidelines in my 'red book' or from the Human Tissue Authority.

I also didn't know I'd end up working sometimes as a prosector in the dissection room at our other campus. A prosection is different from a dissection (the act of cutting something open to study its internal parts), which is what medical students frequently carry out as part of their studies to learn about something they've never seen before. A prosection is the dissection of a cadaver, or part thereof, but it's carried out by an experienced anatomist in order to demonstrate a specific anatomical structure to students. Most dissection rooms will own a series of prosections which the students can observe as they dissect their own donated cadavers – a kind of 3D atlas of body parts. A prosection can be of the cardiorespiratory system, the head and neck, or perhaps a limb. These incredible real-life 'sculptures' created from embalmed donor cadavers illustrate layers of muscle, tendon, fascia, vessels and more. Stored correctly in a preservative such as formalin, these pieces can inform students for years to come. One doesn't need to be 'whole' to help train the doctors and surgeons of the future; fragmented remains are just as useful. Even more interesting was that after years of having to carry out autopsies on fully embalmed cases, the flesh of which becomes as grey and hard as overcooked tuna, I was able to see the newer forms of 'soft-fix' embalming used for donated teaching cadavers.

One example is called the Thiel Method, named after its creator, Austrian anatomist Walter Thiel. He had a 'Eureka!' moment in the butcher's one day when he noticed the preservation of wet-cured ham left the flesh more realistic than the preserved flesh at the Graz Institute. Years later he'd refined his technique, which used a colourless, nearly odourless solution of salts, antiseptic boric acid, ethylene glycol and antifreeze with a very low level of formaldehyde to create incredibly realistic soft cadavers. These newer methods made the dissection a much more authentic experience for the medical students and made me feel like I was right back at home in the post-mortem room.

I was in the Bart's dissection room for the first time one summer, when most of the students had gone home. Some city-based students remained on as paid prosectors through the holiday and the talented anatomy teacher, Carol, had asked if I'd like to join them. She wanted me to help create some prosections for the new term since I had a background in autopsies, and of course I jumped at the chance – I wanted experience with human remains of all types in order to be the most informed I could possibly be. When I was presented with my donor, which was only a head and torso, I began by dissecting out the muscles of the neck, expecting to reveal the sternocleidomastoid – that muscle we APTs cut through when we make our Y-incision.

'Don't go straight for the SCM,' Carol suddenly said, causing me to pause with my scalpel in mid-air. 'Try to reveal the platysma first.'

'What on earth is the platysma?' I'd asked, flummoxed. I had over ten years' experience with human remains but I'd never before heard the term.

Carol was very understanding. 'It's an incredibly superficial muscle that overlaps the SCM,' she explained. 'You won't have seen it in post-mortems. When it's in action it draws down the lower lip and angle of the mouth in expressions like sadness, surprise or horror.' She pointed to her jawbone. 'It also produces a wrinkling of the surface of the skin of the neck and depresses the lower jaw.'

'So it makes us look like Deirdre Barlow from *Coronation Street*?' I asked.

'Haha, exactly!'

Carol started off the process so I could see the tip of this new piece of the human puzzle I had just learned about, then left me to continue with the scalpel. The platysma was no more than two millimetres thick and slightly orange in colour next to the yellow adipose tissue of the neck so it was difficult to differentiate. But I persevered, and I got there: I exposed the whole platysma and suddenly heard a whisper in my ear. It was Carol: 'I knew you'd be good at this.'

I beamed. It was such a strange form of job satisfaction, but now I had created something that would teach other students the position and use of the platysma. Thus the knowledge was being passed on.

I had a lot of fun prosecting. The atmosphere was always wonderful and respectful yet happy because these deceased people were consenting donors who'd usually passed away from natural causes. Even the banter between the other prosectors taught me things I'd never heard of as an APT. One of them, Gavin, came over to my trolley and pointed at the exposed lung of my donor after I'd removed the sternum.

'Look, this one has a lingula.'

Again, I was puzzled by a new anatomical term.

Noticing my face, he continued, 'It's a small, tongue-like structure that sometimes projects from the lower portion of the upper lobe of the left lung.' He flicked it gently with his gloved finger. 'See? It looks like a little puppy tongue.'

'Oh, yeah.' I realised it did on closer inspection. 'And I suppose "lingula" comes from *lingua*, like language.' I thought for a moment, then said, 'But I thought it meant "lips".'

He burst out laughing. 'No, you're talking about labia!'

'Who's talking about labia?' Carol exclaimed as she walked by at just that moment.

I started laughing. '*He* is! He started it!' I pointed at Gavin but we were all laughing by then.

Lips/tongue.

Labia/lingula.

Tomayto/tomahto.

Good old Latin. It reminded me of being in university, studying microbiology with my lab partner Paula, and reading our instructions to swab each other's uvula. 'Right, lie on the floor, Paula, and get your pants down,' I'd said, pretending to misread uvula for vulva. She panicked when she saw me coming at her with a swab, and looked very relieved when she realised I was joking. The uvula, the little drip of flesh that hangs down at the back of the throat which is often mistakenly called the tonsil, is an ample and marginally less X-rated place to obtain various bacteria for study. But it was funny to see the look on Paula's face.

Significantly, the smallest body part removal can change the status of the deceased – something else I didn't learn until I was no longer a full-time APT. Once again, I was lucky enough to be able to film an educational documentary about the autopsy process. I carried out the evisceration of a donor cadaver, alongside a well-known pathologist, with three cameras pointing at me over the course of a few days. In our earlier production meetings it was clear that in the time frame we had to make and air this documentary it would be difficult to receive the perfect donor cadaver from somewhere as small as England. Because the facility we'd be filming in already had a supply contract with a US company – they purchased limbs for surgeons to practise on – it made more sense for the team to use that company. But there was one snag: it's illegal to ship whole bodies for this purpose. The only way it could be done is if one append-age was removed – a hand or a foot, for example. That way, the deceased was classed as a 'body part' but from the right angle would of course look completely whole. A technicality, really.

However, I received a panicked call from our producer one morning a week before filming. 'Carla,' she said, 'they've sent the donor but they've chopped off both her arms. It looks so unsightly – she looks like a turkey!'

'What on earth did they do that—?' I asked, but never got to finish as she interrupted me with, 'But they did also mail us one of her arms. I don't know why they chopped them both off and then mailed one separately. Can you do anything?'

'Are you asking me to come over and sew her arm back on?' I asked. 'Because that's no problem.'

'Would you? Oh my God, you're a lifesaver! I didn't want to ask the question – I thought it sounded weird.'

'It's really not the weirdest question I've been asked,' I assured her – and it wasn't. I regularly receive queries like

'How can I pickle my dead kitten?' and 'Is it possible to taxidermy my wife if she dies?' *If* she dies? To that one I'd replied, 'Well, it's better than doing it when she's alive.'

And so, a couple of days later, I found myself in a high-tech surgical and post-mortem suite, about to reattach the arm of this poor donor woman who'd had it removed in an incredibly unsightly fashion.

'Are you sure you can do this?' asked the producer. 'The edges are all ragged. What did they even use to do it?' She was in a pretty big flap.

'Don't worry,' I said calmly, thinking of all the fragmented cases I'd reconstructed in the past, particularly Railway Man. 'This isn't my first rodeo.'

Once the arm was stitched on, of course it looked heinous, but then I wrapped the join with flesh-coloured sticky bandage. If you squinted your eyes a bit or took a step back you could barely tell it wasn't her own skin. The relief in the air was palpable. Crisis averted.

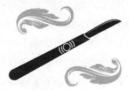

The Victorians, with their elaborate Cult of Mourning, are famous for their use of fragmented human remains in jewellery – mainly hair, but sometimes even teeth and bone. They also used these same body parts as a way to express their love for someone very much alive, whether a child or a partner. The practice became rare after the First World War but it does continue in the modern era. When Lucas Unger proposed to girlfriend Carlee Leifkes in 2015, he did so with a ring made from his wisdom tooth. Prior to that in 2011, Guernsey-based couple Melita and Mike Perrett were married after he proposed with a ring containing a diamond and fragments of bone from his amputated leg. So the Victorian tradition continues, and I think it's lovely that some of the original antique objects, so often mistakenly assumed to be commemorating death, are actually celebrating love.

We fall in love so that in effect we *don't* die: we theoretically live on in the children we're supposed to procreate. Without the threat of looming death, love may not be a priority or instinct.

I would never procreate; I knew that immediately after my miscarriage. None of it had seemed right and I felt broken: I was 'hole' rather than 'whole', keenly aware that where there had been something, there was now nothing. Back then, in that mortuary, at that time, I just couldn't shake the negativity, no matter how much I tried. Then one of my friends from my school days, Gina, came to my rescue with the offer of a week in the South of France – an opportunity to get away from Grey Britain and the imposing walls of my workplace which were closing in on me every day. I only needed the air fare; accommodation was free. I jumped at the chance.

And it was just what I needed. We had long chats on the beach at night beneath the brightest stars I'd ever seen, the sharp edges of my exploding pain blunted by the delicious yet cheap and locally produced red wine. I spent the days languidly in the sun, perhaps drinking more wine than I should – this time ice-cold white in two litre bottles which we'd pick up by cycling five minutes to the local vineyard. Gina went on some excursions – she could speak fluent

French and wanted to explore. I, however, just lay there on our veranda, burning in the hot French sun, partly wondering if I could incinerate away the feeling of being tainted since excessive bathing hadn't been working. I was pretty drunk. It was a bad plan.

One evening we headed out to the fairground and I was dizzy with the noise and the music and the lights. It was a surreal experience, as though I was dreaming. After so many quiet days the noise seemed tempestuous in my head, but somehow challenging. I wanted to feel something other than what I'd been feeling for too long, so I begged Gina to come with me on ride after ride. Sometimes spinning horizontally, sometimes vertically, sometimes swinging like a pendulum. Then, finally, I told her I wanted to go on the rollercoaster. Maybe an adrenalin rush would get the endorphins going and fix my brain? The rickety apparatus didn't necessarily instil any confidence in us but, truth be told, it didn't scare me either.

It swerved and ascended and descended and went upside down, and I did something I'd never, ever done on a rollercoaster before: I let go.

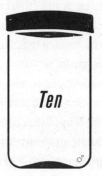

Ten

Reconstruction:
'All the King's Men'

> You may see a cup of tea fall off of a table and break into pieces on the floor. But you will never see the cup gather itself back together and jump back on the table ... The increase of disorder, or entropy, is what distinguishes the past from the future.
>
> —*Stephen Hawking,*
> A Brief History of Time

Of course, I didn't die on that rollercoaster – I was belted in. But that night taught me something about my frame of mind at the time and I knew it had to stop. I had to move on.

*

I don't know what had caused my Railway Man to jump in front of an oncoming train, but I had an inkling of what his mindset must have been like. One thing was certain: once he had done it, there was no going back. Time would not rewind. The spectators at the station would not see him consolidate in an arcing red and pink implosion and then land on the train platform, safe and complete. I wondered what had gone through his mind as he leaped. Did he regret it and become filled with terror? Was he grateful for the imminent sensation of peace and relief he had so craved? Or was there time for neither of those things before he was struck by the train's relentless steel?

I had plenty of time to wonder about it because I had decided to spend hours reconstructing this suicide victim entirely, to do the best I could to piece him back together. The Coroner's Officer hadn't expected his family to be able to view him. Unlike the brief autopsy, the reconstruction process took me four hours, but every minute was worth it to hear the voice on the end of the phone say 'Sorry, what?' in response to the statement I had just made.

'I said, his family can view this afternoon, or tomorrow if they like.'

'I don't understand.' The Coroner's Officer was clearly baffled. 'I thought he was in pieces. The BTP and the recovery team said there was no way he'd be viewable.'

'He *was* in pieces,' I explained, 'but part of our job is to do the best we can to make sure the deceased is in a respectable and dignified state. In this case, actually viewable.'

'Okaaay,' she said, and I could hear the scepticism in her voice. 'You're going to have to talk me through this one.'

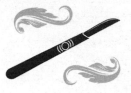

Using the phrase 'all the King's men' from 'Humpty Dumpty' is not meant to be facetious. Much like the superficially nonsensical *Alice in Wonderland* is said to contain mathematical references such as the concepts of 'limit' and 'inverse relationships', 'Humpty Dumpty' is often used to represent the Second Law of Thermodynamics. Earlier, when I was describing the ecosystem of a decaying cadaver, I mentioned the First Law of Thermodynamics, which states that energy cannot be created or destroyed, it can only change form. The Second Law states that 'the total entropy of an isolated system always increases over time', entropy in this context meaning disorder or chaos. In the rhyme, after the unfortunate egg falls and is shattered into pieces, 'all the King's horses and all the King's men couldn't put Humpty together again'. The inability to restore poor Mr Dumpty to the way he was before his fall is a representation of this principle.

This law describes perfectly the reconstruction of the deceased after a post-mortem examination too. APTs are not embalmers and don't use cosmetics and high-tech superficial methods to reconstruct a patient; they have to begin from the very inside, as though the deceased were a completely cracked egg, and do their best to make them whole again.

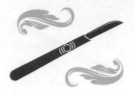

Just after hosing the dissection bench and surfaces down, I threw a bucket of warm water and disinfectant over the stainless-steel bench and let it soak for a while. Then I moved to my case, Railway Man. When washing the deceased we'd use the hose too, but the aim was to keep it gentle, to try to avoid blood and tiny particles of tissue being splashed all over the floor and equipment, and creating an aerosol of minuscule blood drops which could be inhaled. The post-mortem tray is usually on a slight incline, with the deceased's head at the top, meaning that the water flows down the body and tray, then out through a plughole leading to a sink at the deceased's feet. It might seem strange, this washing of the dead, as though they're a car or dishes in a restaurant, but in reality, with a gentle touch, it's not too disconcerting. In one hand I'd hold the trigger of the hose like a pistol, and in the other I'd hold a sponge soaked in a mild, foaming sanitiser. I'd clean the blood off constantly throughout the procedure, not only because it's mortuary best practice and more dignified for the patient, but also because it stops the blood coagulating on the skin which makes it far more difficult to remove later. The soap and blood mixing together would form a familiar pink lather that slid down the arms and legs of the decedent and swirled around the plughole. It was familiar because I saw it every day, and now, when I wash my red hair, the pink suds that fill the bath and embark on a similar spiralling journey look exactly the same. I feel like I'm straight back in the post-mortem room.

The part that was disconcerting was hosing the face. Even the gentlest of spray over the mouth and open eyes would cause me to expect a flinch; to expect the eyes to close reflexively against the onslaught, and the head to turn away. But, thankfully, that never happened. The water would just splash across the half-exposed eyeballs and drip into the open mouth of the deceased. I didn't like it when small globules of debris or fatty yellow adipose tissue became caught in the teeth and against the gums. I couldn't just spray harder into the mouth – that didn't seem right. Instead, I used to brush their teeth with a proper toothbrush.

I'm not sure how many of my colleagues ever noticed that.

Once the patient had had a first clean down, I'd begin the reconstruction. First, the head. Since the hair was wet it was easier to comb in the same way I did earlier while making the incision: half of the hair up and over the face, half down the back of the neck. Unlike perinatal cases, whose brains are huge in relation to the body, the brains of the adult deceased do not go back into the head. This would be impossible because the brain is such a soft organ – I described it as a 'mousse' earlier – and the face has so many natural orifices it would be unsanitary. Instead, I dried the base of the skull with blue roll then took a huge wad of fresh white cotton wool and moulded it into the approximate size and shape of the brain. I placed this into the empty skull cavity, for two reasons: first, it gave shape to the head by allowing me to place the calvarium on top and keep it stable; second, the absorbent nature meant it would soak up any fluid which might leak from the foramen magnum, or any fluids I'd missed with the blue roll.

With the skull reconstructed, I'd smooth the temporal muscles back into place then pull the scalp over so that one side of the incision joined the other side at the back of the head, with just a small gap between. Then I'd sew, using my pre-prepared needle and PM twine, in the exact same way I'd made the earlier cut with the scalpel – from right to left. I'd push my S-shaped needle up and under the upper flap of scalp, exactly in the middle where the yellow adipose tissue and even the bulbs of the hair roots could be seen. Then I'd push it down and under the lower flap in the same place. Up and under, down and under, and on and on, until I had created a neat seam which resembled the stitches on a baseball. We actually call it baseball stitch.

After that, I'd dry out the body cavity with more blue roll or a clean sponge and place more fresh, white cotton wool into the pelvis. This replaces the bladder and pelvic organs and again absorbs any fluids before they can escape through the body's natural orifices. I'd add more cotton wool to the neck for the same reason, as well as to give the neck some shape back, sometimes even forming a little Adam's apple for the men. This meant that every single organ from the deceased was placed into biodegradable clear bags – the viscera bags. They're made for this specific purpose – we don't use bin bags or clinical waste bags. The bag, neatly tied, can be placed into the empty body cavity, and then the sternum, which was previously removed to access the heart and lungs, is placed on top. This, again, gives the patient a natural shape. I'd bring the two main flaps of skin together and stitch the incision in exactly the same way as I'd made that too, from top to bottom, using the same baseball stitch.

If I'd had to remove vitreous from the eyes of my case, I'd

inject saline into them to maintain the intraocular pressure, which would give them back their spherical shape. If I'd taken out false teeth, they'd go back in now. The face would often look more at peace after an autopsy than before. I'd once again wash the body completely and shampoo the hair to remove any grease or residual body fluids. Sometimes I'd clean the fingernails, and if any sores continued to ooze, for example ulcers or sites of medical intervention, I'd wrap them in an absorbent bandage or cover them in a large plaster. Once dried with a towel and placed into a temporary, single-use shroud the deceased looked clean, complete and at peace.

But the Second Law of Thermodynamics is in action. It's not possible for us to put every single organ back into its original position by stitching them in place like pieces of a jigsaw, and it's not possible for us to refill the veins and arteries with the blood of the deceased – this will have disappeared down the drain and entered the sewage system like every other type of waste produced by the population. Quite simply, we cannot put Humpty Dumpty back together again. No one can.

What we can try to do is such a good job of it that the deceased looks much better and much more cared for after the process of a post-mortem than before it.

My Railway Man was more complicated than this. I had to use the same baseball stitch to secure every severed and partly severed limb: the two hands (at the wrists), one leg (just below the knee) and one foot (at the ankle). I then had to do the same thing all around his waist as he had been practically split into two. What I was left with really did resemble a crude Frankenstein's monster – as though I'd taken various body parts out of the limb bin and stitched them to a head and torso in order to make my own 'Adam'. But after I'd wrapped flesh-toned bandage around each join, these ugly indicators of a violent death were hidden. He looked so much better.

I explained this to the Coroner's Officer on the phone.

'How long did that take?' she asked, incredulous.

'About four hours or so. But it was the head that was a lot more hard work.'

In fact, it had taken me nearly an extra hour to fill the cavity with as much cotton wool as possible then glue some fragments of skull to it with superglue, in what I guessed were the correct anatomical positions. I'd then wrapped the whole head in a white bandage, taking it further down on the left side to cover most of the damaged tissue.

'He looks a bit like Mr Bump, OK?' I warned the Coroner's Officer. 'But he is perfectly viewable – you can see his face quite clearly.'

'Amazing. I'll let the family know,' she said.

I was pleased for the family and I was pleased for him, but I couldn't stop thinking of the decision he'd made, from which there was no going back, and how I'd diced with such a decision, and how this case had come just at the right time to teach me a valuable lesson.

Often APTs will say they do what they do for the families of the dead, and of course this is very often true. However, it's also a way for them to explain why they do a job which can seem so odd to most people. It normalises it. It can be a way to receive some positive reinforcement for the hard work that goes into assisting at a post-mortem, then reconstructing the deceased; a chance for them to be thanked by someone. We all need that encouragement, whatever job we do.

What I find odd is how few admit that they also do this job for the dead themselves. When I reconstructed the anorexic dentist, no one came to see him or claim him, yet I carried out my reconstruction duties anyway, even going above and beyond what some mortuaries require. This wasn't for the family; it was for him. I didn't expect a 'thank you, he looks wonderful' from anyone, although of course sometimes, like in the case of my Railway Man, I did receive that type of praise. In general, we APTs thoroughly enjoy working to the best of our ability, most of us like to do as much as we can for the families, and our main purpose is to provide the dead with some dignity as they pass through our care.

Why, then, are some APTs so quick to censor their activities by frowning upon honest accounts of autopsies in the media or photographs of the procedure released by artists like Sue Fox and Cathrine Ertmann; or by not allowing people to view any part of the post-mortem process (unless they absolutely must); or by euphemising their job as something they do 'for the living'? If they can't even admit what their job actually consists of, if they keep the profession shrouded in secrecy, if they don't illustrate that they are human beings too and that they can have a sense of humour and still be a good pathology technician, then how are the general public supposed to assume those things? It's as though the profession is creating its own taboo on the dead.

I've since researched secrecy and transparency in all aspects of the death professions: mortuary work, funeral work, skeletal excavation, public display of human remains and more.

It is often fragments of the human being that I tend to focus on, given my position as technical curator of a pathology collection, but I also keep up to date with studies on mortality salience (our understanding of death), death theory and constantly changing legislation regarding the dead. Back then, during that difficult time, I needed something to focus on in my evenings, so I began to read more of my old books and acquire some of the classics such as *The Denial of Death* by Ernest Becker and *The American Way of Death* by Jessica Mitford. I connected with people on social media who felt death shouldn't be kept behind closed doors, quietly following the 'Death Positive' movement revived by an insightful and humorous mortician from the US, Caitlin Doughty, who wanted death to be talked about in the open; to do for mortality what the earlier 'Sex Positive' movement had done for sexuality.

I began to form my own theories as I learned about the benefits of open communication about death. After all, it was secrecy which led to the organ retention scandal, and an attitude of 'tell them as little as they need to know' which caused so many problems further down the line. I attended conferences in different cities and met up with some of the people I'd been chatting with online. At one conference I heard of a fascinating study called 'Bones without Barriers', which encompassed everything I was trying to argue for. In a nutshell, a team of archaeologists erected screens around their excavation site and began to exhume skeletal remains. The local residents weren't happy: they wondered what was going on 'behind the screens' and in the absence of any actual knowledge they feared the worst, imagining the excavation to be a desecration of people's graves and that there was no real reason for it to be done. The insinuation was, if they weren't up to no good then why hide what they were doing? After a certain amount of time the second part of the study commenced. This involved removing all the screens and allowing the general public to approach and ask the archaeological team questions; in some cases they were even allowed to handle the bones. Questionnaires revealed that the public had been much happier about the excavation during the screenless phase: they understood the procedure more and were interested in what was going on rather than offended by it.

The study opened my eyes to a world out there that might still involve me using my skills but being able to communicate about it. I didn't quite know what I wanted to do yet, but I could feel all my own fragmented pieces coming back together again as I began to focus on that aim. I was tired of being in a profession in which I was told 'You're not supposed to talk about your day unless it's with a long-term partner or a parent. Don't discuss it with just anyone.' I was tired of the fear of God being put into me about making a mistake because if I did 'it'll be another Alder Hey'. I was tired of even hearing that phrase!

The paperwork increased, but I felt like it wasn't relevant; it wasn't progressing my or many APTs' general aims. I would have liked to attend quarterly APT meet-ups and contribute more to our organisation, the Association for Anatomical Pathology Technologists (AAPT), but instead I was responsible for things like ensuring that the whole pathology team, including all the doctors, were carrying out their Manual Handling and Health and Safety training. I may as well have been working in clinical governance.

Still, I took it all on board as 'experience', but even though I increased my hours I couldn't quite keep on top of it all. Then I realised another reason why I'd wanted to stay with Railway Man and reconstruct him no matter how long it took: I had wanted to stay in the little High Risk PM room. I didn't want to come out and work in the office. I wanted to do the thing I'd wanted to do since I was a child, the one thing that never seems to get mentioned by other APTs – I wanted to work with the dead.

That was when I knew I had to leave.

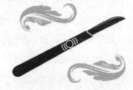

Whilst looking for other jobs, I made sure I spent as much time as I could in the post-mortem rooms. There was always something to be learned from veterans of pathology like Professor St Clare and many of the other consultant pathologists who would come on a rota system to carry out the day's cases. Not all mortuaries work the same way so I made sure I was registered on a database for locum APTs so that I could use my annual leave, or time between jobs, to work in other facilities. And I did look for managerial jobs in other mortuaries because smaller (particularly local authority) ones tend to have a lot less paperwork and the manager will carry out more autopsies. There were other death professions I was looking into as well – 'there's more than one way to skin a cat', they say. In fact, there's more than one way to skin a human being. I found this out as part of my ever-expanding research . . .

One afternoon, we had a phone call which Tina answered. As she listened to the voice on the other end I could see her looking more and more forlorn.

'What is it, Teen?' I asked, after she'd put the receiver down. 'Last-minute viewing or something?'

'No, it was the tissue bank. There's a skin and bone donor here and they want to do it this afternoon.'

'Why is that a problem?' I asked, curious. I'd never seen it done before.

'Because it takes *for ever*,' she groaned. 'I'm on call but I'm supposed to go to a meeting with Juan and the clinical governance team. The tissue people can't do it unsupervised – someone needs to be in the office, able to pop in and out of the PM room.'

'I'll stay with them,' I offered. I probably wouldn't stay in the office, I'd go in and watch the process.

'Really? You'd do that?' asked Tina.

'Of course! I want to see how they do it, anyway. Don't worry about it – go to your meeting.' It seems Tina was way more cut out for the clinical governance life than I was.

So, an hour later, I was happily ensconced in the post-mortem room with the technicians from NHSBT Tissue Services explaining the procedure they were about to carry out. They were both so cheerful! Johnny, plump, with brown hair and about thirty years old, was happy to answer all of my questions because the younger girl he was with, Sonya, was his trainee. She was able to learn some new things during the discussion, too.

'So you had to come and do this today – it couldn't be put off until tomorrow?' I asked as I removed the donor from the fridge. 'I mean, not that it's a problem – I just wondered.'

As we moved the donor into the PM room, Johnny explained, 'We have up to forty-eight hours to remove most tissues but if the donor has ticked this consent box' – he pointed to a specific part of the paperwork – 'then we really want to come and get them as soon as possible, certainly within twenty-four hours if we can. They're more likely to be successfully transplanted if they're harvested sooner.'

'Harvested' is the technical term for removal of any tissue from a cadaver in this context. The tissues he was referring to were skin and bone in this instance, and anyone can tick the box to donate them after their death. (Tendons and heart valves can only be donated by those under sixty years of age). However, just like with other organs, it doesn't necessarily mean the tissue will be used: it can depend on factors like whether or not an infectious disease is present or whether it's too damaged by injury. Of course, decomposition is a factor, too. That's why there needs to be an excess number of donors out there, more than we actually need.

'A lot of people don't know that even if they're alive they can donate skin,' Johnny added, slipping into his PPE. 'You know, if someone loses a lot of weight and has excess skin surgically removed?'

I hadn't even known that. As usual, I was just focused on the dead. 'That's a really good idea – I'd never have thought of that,' I answered as I watched him open his 'harvesting kit'.

He pulled out an instrument that looked like a large stainless-steel razor with a clunkier head. It had a cable attached to it, and he plugged it in.

'This is a Dermatome – it's like a big razor with an oscillating blade,' he said as he examined the deceased to see which skin parts were best to harvest. Obviously nothing visible that would alter reconstruction – mainly his thighs. The Dermatome buzzed, and because it was electric it enabled him to remove rectangles of skin of a uniform size and thickness, unlike manual ones which he told me could be a bit more irregular.

It was so incredible watching him remove these long swathes of skin from the deceased, the hair still attached and glowing under the fluorescent lights, before handing them to Sonya to be placed into special packaging.

'What happens to them afterwards?' I asked, utterly rapt.

'Once they've been treated they get placed on a meshing device which basically turns them into nets.'

It's these nets of skin you see grafted on to individuals who've been extensively injured. Common uses for them are burns, skin infections and bedsores or ulcers that haven't healed well. Had my anorexic dentist survived his septicaemia he probably would have needed grafts like this.

As Johnny worked and chatted he made the procedure sound so modern, with his electric tools and sentences peppered with the words 'cryopreserved', 'irradiated' and 'antibiotic incubation', but accounts of skin grafting have been found as early as 2500 years ago, in India.

But there's another use for this cadaver skin, something I didn't know about until a couple of years later. I mentioned I have a facial condition called Parry-Romberg Syndrome, which is quite rare. I talk about this and any other health issues I've had simply to illustrate that even though I work in pathology that doesn't give me a 'get out of jail free' card when it comes to my health; we're all people, prone to the effects of pathology's capricious nature. I'd love it if my decision to work in this field had involved me making a dark pact with the Grim Reaper to ensure me and my loved ones immunity from death and disease, but unfortunately that's not the case. It's a shame really. I'd like to do something dramatic like sign a scroll of parchment in blood ... or would it in fact be a scroll of skin, removed using an infernal antique Dermatome? We'll never know.

Anyway, my particular condition, also known as hemifacial atrophy, was caused by physical trauma – I wasn't born with it – and, among some other more serious symptoms, it makes my face asymmetrical. The tissues basically dissolve on one side. Every year or two, like a car having an MOT, I go into hospital for surgery to even out my facial structure. My surgeon had previously removed those pieces of my fascia and my own body fat but they too had dissolved after they'd been implanted in my face for a while. The next attempt, he'd said with some gravity, was to use 'Alloderm', which was *cadaver skin*. When he uttered that phrase he looked at me as though he was expecting a peal of thunder.

'OK,' I said, unperturbed.

'It may well be more stable,' he added, so quickly I assumed he was worried I'd change my mind. 'I would have mentioned it sooner, but I didn't want to scare you off with the idea.'

'Oh, for goodness sake, Mr Mahmoud, I work in a *mortuary*! I don't mind a bit of cadaver skin in my face!'

And that was how I came to be the Bride of Frankenstein, physically reconstructed from the parts of the generous dead.

Back in the post-mortem room, Tissue Services were now hard at work removing the bones from our donor, namely the femur, tibia and fibula in the legs. This involved creating a deep incision into the flesh of the leg, much deeper than an APT would usually need to go, and cutting right through the fascia, which was amazing for me to watch considering I had half of my leg fascia in my face but had never actually seen it. The bones were replaced with silicon rods of the same dimensions so the legs didn't end up 'floppy'. 'They used to use sawn-off wooden mop handles before these, you know,' Johnny told me. It made sense. A lot of things used to be made of wood.

The procedure was similar to when we APTs made an incision into the deceased's calf muscles to check for deep vein thrombosis (DVT), a condition many are familiar with because of its association with flying (though it's more to do with being immobile for long periods of time). If a clot or coagulated blood embolism forms in the leg vein and part of it breaks off, it may circulate through the body and end up in the lungs, causing a fatal pulmonary embolism. If the pathologist found such an embolism, also called a PE, I'd then inspect the muscles of the calf to ascertain its origin. Sometimes it was visible to the naked eye which calf contained the DVT as it was slightly swollen, but other times I'd just have to delve. The difference is I'd be searching in the vessels of the calf muscles and not incising quite as deep into the bone. But despite the difference in depth, Johnny reconstructed the incision in exactly the same way as we did.

'Oh look, he's an eye donor as well,' Sonya pointed out, seemingly pleased that she'd noticed this on the form.

'I can remove eyes!' I exclaimed, like a kid on the front row in the classroom. 'Well, I have a certificate ... I haven't actually done it yet,' I admitted.

'Do you want to retrieve these?' Johnny offered. 'Sonya has to watch anyway – she hasn't done the course yet.'

'Oh God, no, I can't remember how I did it now.'

'Well, how about I do the first one, you watch, then you do the second?'

I was shocked. 'You'd trust me? What if I ruin it?'

'You eviscerate *whole bodies*, don't you?' he pointed out. 'I'm sure you can manage one eye.'

Fair point.

So, after observing Johnny deftly remove the left eye, drop it in a container of sterile solution with a muted 'plop' and place it straight on ice, I took a fresh scalpel and removed my first eye. To do so I had to open the eyelids with metal retractors as he had done, creating a slightly harrowing tableau which reminded me of *A Clockwork Orange*. But it meant I could access and slice through the conjunctival muscles and optic nerve with the disposable scalpel, as easy as a knife through butter. Within seconds the right eye was also on ice and ready to go to one of two main tissue banks in the UK, where it could be stored for up to thirty-eight days. I reconstructed the socket by fashioning a spherical wad of cotton wool the same dimensions as an eyeball and then placing on a smooth plastic eye cap for roundness. Once re-dressed the man looked exactly as he had before. The fact that these tissues had been harvested wasn't obvious at all – he was perfectly reassembled.

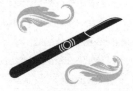

The bodies of the deceased who were severely decomposed – the 'decomps' – were reconstituted in the exact same way as everybody else. There was no way they would usually be viewed by family members – our current aversion to decayed cadavers in the West has made it highly unlikely. On the odd occasion when family members insisted on viewing their decomposed dead – and by 'insist' I mean literally refuse to leave the building without seeing them – in some mortuaries we had to make them sign a waiver. The form basically stated that we had informed the next of kin of the condition of the deceased – the colour, the smell, the fact that this will not look like the person they remember – and they had accepted that and were still prepared to go in.

The decomposed will also under no circumstances be embalmed because they're too decayed. The fragile veins would be unable to withstand such strong chemicals and the colour changes I've already described can't be altered, either. But that's not the point. We reconstruct the dead for the dead. The decayed dead deserve the same treatment as everyone else so we still place the organ pulp into a viscera bag, still fill the skull with cotton wool and close the scalp, and still attempt to stitch the leathery skin of mummified remains back together, even if their desiccation and shrunken state means there'll be a gap. We then sprinkle an absorbent, scented powder into the bag, zip it up, and usually place that into another bag. And then another one. And if there's someone around to pay for a funeral they will have a closed-casket ceremony regardless of whether they're buried or cremated.

The dead can't be reconstructed perfectly, and perhaps that's the point – they're not supposed to be. Although we in the West only see decomposing cadavers in horror films and computer games, that certainly wasn't always the case.

Thirteenth-century Buddhists practised their Nine Cemetery Contemplations, or Maranasati meditation, with the help of artwork depicting all aspects of human decomposition. These pieces, known as *kusozu*, were a visual aid to assist the Buddhists' reflection on the various phases of death and were still popular in the nineteenth century, and in recent times I have had Buddhists ask to view my museum specimens for the same purpose. The ultimate aim of Maranasati is to appreciate mortality and to accept the changing nature of all things, therefore increasing mindfulness. As these decomposing corpses tended to start out as beautiful courtesans in the artwork, there was also an element of enforcing chastity among the monks during these meditations, the idea being that her outside form may be beautiful, yet underneath it all she will rot and decay like everyone else.

It's the same lesson I took from this multitude of decomposed decedents. It's very difficult to hold on to the idea of the importance or significance of the minutiae of the day when faced, literally, with a decomposing human. The Buddhists teach impermanence, the notion that all existence is transient or in a constant state of flux. That transience is there before your very eyes in the changing state of the deceased – it exists in a liminal space, not really dead and not really alive. The process is nature's great leveller. The Greeks and Romans slept in tombs to receive inspiration from the dead, and the same lesson was taught in the West via medieval art, whether paintings or sculptures, which showed skeletons crawling with what they called 'worms' as well as other insects. The painting *Allegory of Death* by the circle of Juan de Valdés Leal is very typical of the era. It depicts a skeleton, somewhere between advanced decay and dry remains, reclining with its guts hanging out and beetles munching at exposed leg bones. Their 'transitional nature' – deceased yet teeming with life – means that models of rotting carcasses, popular in the later medieval era, came to be known as transis. A transi can be lifesize and carved in stone or tiny and made from ivory; either way, it is a memento mori, a reminder that death comes for us all and decay is natural.

At the end of the seventeenth century in Europe, meditation on the decay of the body within the tomb, with as much detail as possible, was recommended as a spiritual exercise. Around 1667, the manual *L'uomo al Punto di Morti* ('Man at the Point of Death') by Jesuit writer Daniello Bartoli suggested this as a means to understand death. It included a chapter entitled 'The tomb a school able to make even the mad wise: we enter therein to hear a lesson of moral and Christian philosophy'. The wax bust known as La Donna Scandalosa, created at the turn of the eighteenth century in Naples, depicts a beautiful woman's face and chest just visible through soil. She is covered in 'worms' and even has a rat gnawing at her breast. These images and writings were visual reminders of that famous verse:

Remember me as you pass by,
As you are now, so once was I,
As I am now, so you must be,
Prepare for death and follow me.

Those who lived during times of pestilence and torture were almost transgressively intimate with the decomposing corpse in a way we in the clinical and airbrushed West are not. But a small minority are beginning to protest against that hidden, antiseptic world of dying and instead embrace a more natural approach to death and decomposition. 'Green funerals' are becoming increasingly popular. Funeral directors are discouraging the use of chemical embalming and coffins made from non-biodegradable material. Wicker and even cardboard coffins are being suggested instead, and natural or 'woodland' burials in sustainable land rather than non-environmentally-friendly churchyard burials and cremation. Suddenly, Munch's quote 'From my rotting body, flowers shall grow and I am in them and that is eternity' is becoming more of a reality. Why spend so much time artificially reconstructing the dead when our natural fate is to be recycled and, in whatever way you look at it, 'reborn'?

The Buddhists understand impermanence. They understand that things change. So we can fragment, we can fall to pieces, and we can *let* ourselves do so, without the intervention of chemical and physical stabilisers. But, regardless of religious beliefs, we will in some way be reconstituted – a fate meant to befall us all.

In the end we come full circle.

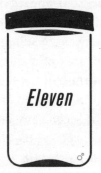

Eleven

Chapel of Rest: 'Sister Act'

Almost everyone has or will experience getting
dumped in their lifetime. Unless, of course,
you're a nun. Jesus can't dump nuns.

—Jenny McCarthy,
Love, Lust & Faking It: The Naked Truth
About Sex, Lies, and True Romance

I woke up at 5.15 a.m., and not naturally. I'd needed to use the
alarm on my phone, which defeated the object of being here,
really. The idea was to be secluded, alone, undistracted by the
trivial things. I wanted my phone to stay *off*.

Note to self: buy a travel alarm clock.

I also did not want to get out of bed. The basic sheets I'd
climbed under in this small room the night before hadn't

felt particularly luxurious, but now, with the heat of my body from a night's sleep cocooning me in comfiness, it felt like the best bed in the world. The air outside was so cold on my face it made me want to snuggle in deeper. But then I remembered the wall-mounted fan heater above my bed. I reached out of the warmth of the sheets for the pull string of the heater with lightning speed, like a viper striking at its prey. Within a split second my arm was back where it belonged beneath the covers, as the room began to fill with a gentle whirring and balmy air. I nestled back into my pillow.

I must have stayed in that pleasant state for around fifteen minutes, somewhere between waking and sleeping, until I heard singing gradually amplifying and I reluctantly opened my eyes. I knew it must be five thirty because Nocturns had begun. The gentle, sweet sound of the nuns' hymn was too hard to resist. Like Scooby Doo transported through the air alongside the smell of some delicious food, I floated through the convent and accessed the Chapel through a special door, one which only guests could use. This entrance led to a small balcony that overlooked the interior of the church: the main door to the right which admitted people all day, the rows of pews and therefore the tops of various heads dotted here and there, and the altar on which the monstrance holding the Blessed Sacrament (the holy 'wafer') was glowing like a golden halo as the sun rose through the windows. I could only see one nun at the altar and she was kneeling in Adoration of the Blessed Sacrament, completely motionless – she could have been embalmed and propped there. Certainly she reminded me of the increasingly common practice of 'lifelike' embalming which had occurred several times in the past year. These *muerto parado*, or 'standing dead', were created by an enterprising undertaker who preserved the deceased in lifelike postures after death, even positioning them so that they could attend their own funerals and eternally carry out their favourite pastimes. An eighty-three-year-old New Orleans socialite was posed with a pink feather boa and a glass of champagne; a Puerto Rican man was placed on his favourite motorcycle; one woman was propped up with a beer in one hand and a menthol cigarette in the other.

But there was no smoking or drinking here, alive or dead. This was a convent that practised 'Perpetual Adoration of the Blessed Sacrament', which meant that someone had to be in front of that wafer, on their knees, 24/7; sometimes members of the congregation and sometimes nuns. There was a sign-up sheet at the front of the church with a timetable on it and any devotional gaps not filled by worshippers were taken by the inhabitants of the small convent. The reason I couldn't see the singing nuns and only hear them is that they were a cloistered community and spent as much of their time as possible out of sight, somewhere to the side of the main altar. This was no upbeat Gospel Choir song and dance – it was first thing in the morning, yet their gentle, ethereal harmony was like a lullaby trying to entice me back to sleep. I closed my eyes and sagged against my chair but I didn't fall asleep. I let the sound wash over and through me. I tried to make my mind blank – something I'd been practising a lot – and instead just absorb the melody. During the quieter parts of the refrain I could hear the birds singing outside, their dawn chorus joining with that of the nuns.

I was completely at peace.

Every mortuary facility should have a place for patients to be viewed, in peace and privacy, if possible. However, some mortuaries are too small or too busy so funeral directors always have places for viewings, with larger firms having several rooms for multiple viewings. In all of these buildings the Chapel of Rest was the place in which viewings would occur. I say *was* because in our current, secular society we now call these areas Viewing Rooms. It's less specific to certain religions so it's less offensive, but the phrase still doesn't have the same sense of peace that comes with 'Chapel of Rest'. Peace is important for families viewing their deceased loved ones, but it had also always been important for me. From my very first days dozing contentedly at J. Ellwoods and Sons Funeral Directors in Worthing, via my time trying to obtain some distance from the Terror Trio, right through to me spending my lunch breaks in the tiny hospital church at St Martin's after my miscarriage, these 'chapels' had been my sanctuary. I'm not a religious person, at least not in the traditional sense, and I embrace all forms of worship as well as respect people's decisions not to worship at all. However, the solitude and silence of these solemn places – whether the magnificent Hagia Sophia Mosque in Istanbul or that tiny yet phenomenal bone-strewn church, the Sedlec Ossuary, near Prague – have always been a comfort to me. I've often wondered if one of the reasons I wanted to work with the deceased was because I craved the silence, the stillness, the sense of something sacred.

I was once asked in an interview 'If you weren't an anatomical pathology technologist, what would you be?' and on impulse I replied, 'A nun.' I remember the writer of the feature practically spluttering down the phone, 'I have never in all my years heard *that* one before!'

Of course, I could never really be a nun – I love cocktails and silk nightgowns and red lipstick too much. And I knew that for sure after having had a short trial, while I was trying to gain a little bit of peace by proxy to take away. Just like the deceased, those who choose to be 'consecrated religious' exist at the periphery of both the mundane and the awesome.

Most mortuary viewing rooms have a comfortable sofa and sometimes chairs; they have soft carpets and muted lighting, and often fresh flowers. There isn't usually a piece of furniture for the deceased in the room because they will be prepped outside it on a trolley, usually in the fridge room – a 'transition' or 'orange' area, depending on where you are. Only after prepping will they make their short journey into the womb-like comfort of the viewing chamber.

It's a stark contrast. The fridge room's fluorescent lights are just as unforgiving to the deceased as they are the living (consider your reflection when confronted with industrial lights in public bathrooms: the horror ... the *horror*). But in this situation it's helpful for us APTs because seeing the decedent in stark light at their very worst means we can attempt to rectify every detail so the next of kin can view with peace of mind. We aren't embalmers, though, and just as with reconstruction our techniques are limited. We don't use cosmetics, and try to keep to minimally invasive methods to hide imperfections. For example, if the decedent's mouth is gaping like Ghostface from the *Scream* films we avoid suturing them shut. Instead, we place extra pillows behind the head so that the chin rests on the chest and naturally closes the mouth. If that doesn't work, we can use chin collars: thin pale plastic devices shaped like two rounded triangles connected at an obtuse angle. These press on the chest and push up the jaw at the same time but due to their colour and opacity they can barely be seen. Very often, we have to take forceps and place pieces of cotton wool into the nostrils to absorb fluids. It can't be helped – if the deceased is 'purging' from their nose there is no way we can allow a viewer to experience that. Cotton wool is also handy for closing eyelids which won't stay shut: we take tiny pieces and place them in the eye before closing – nowhere near as large as the pieces I'd use in reconstruction – and the friction stops the serous (slippery) inner eyelid membrane from sliding back up the eyeball. I know, I know, it doesn't sound pleasant, but after viewing it can be removed and no damage is done. The eyes can still be removed for corneal transplant and vitreous can still be aspirated. Consider instead the embalmers' apparatus, the 'eye cap', which is a plastic half-sphere covered in spikes which hook into the eyelid skin forcing them shut, never to be removed again. We do what we can with very little, and ultimately it means a decedent is left with a natural look of 'gentle repose' and nothing that we've done is permanent or invasive. That, as APTs, is our brief.

Why do we carry out these viewings, particularly if we have little space, time and equipment for them? Sometimes, it is simply so that the deceased can be identified before they undergo a post-mortem – and that's another reason we change the face as little as possible: we need them to be familiar to the person doing the ID. Other times, it really is a case of a family or friend or partner needing to see their loved one – needing to know they are dead – before they can move on with funeral arrangements and paperwork. It's therefore not possible for us to recommend they wait until the deceased is at the funeral director's because without this validation a funeral may never happen. We have to help some people work through their denial of the death, particularly if it was sudden.

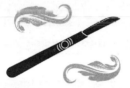

In the 1994 Quentin Tarantino film *Pulp Fiction*, the protagonists, Vincent and Jules, retrieve a briefcase for gangster Marsellus Wallace. When the briefcase is opened using a numeric combination we, the viewer, only see a golden glow reflected on to Vincent's face, never the actual contents. This has led to a lot of speculation about what the case contained: gold bullion, a small nuclear device, Elvis's gold suit or something else? The most prevalent theory is that the case contained the soul of Wallace who had sold it to the Devil and wanted it returned – a theory backed by the '666' combination of the briefcase and biblical passages peppered through the film thanks to the articulate and religious hitman Jules.

Vincent's experience happened to me one morning when I opened one of the fridges at St Martin's and was bathed in a gentle silver light. This was unusual because body fridges aren't like the ones we have at home: they don't have a light in them for us to be able to reach to the back and grab a snack. They're always dark. I was confused for a moment, blinking against the light and wondering, 'Am I seeing a soul leaving a body? Is it a Guardian Angel? Could it all be *real*?' But eventually my eyes adjusted and I realised the light was being emitted from a white body bag. Intrigued, I opened the bag and inside it I found a torch, the light of which was much stronger now that it was uncovered. Somebody had turned on a torch and placed it in the body bag overnight with the deceased.

'What on earth is *that*?' I heard, suddenly. Roxy, a young spunky APT with the most enviable figure I'd ever seen in real life, was halfway down the fridge room teaching our new trainee, Kathy, the process of measuring and checking bodies. She had seen the light – not spiritually, but literally – and started to make her way towards me, asking Kathy to 'Bring that register, will you?'

'It's a torch, but I'm not quite sure why,' I said as I racked my brain trying to remember why this would be in here. When studying to be an APT it's imperative that we learn about various religions and their death customs so we can fully respect different families' wishes. This is why, over the years, I had become more and more familiar with different paths and begun to ask questions of religion and existence myself. It seemed to be a part of advancing through my career, just something that came up on a daily basis. As a Senior it would look pretty poor if I couldn't explain this unusual and rare death ritual to the other staff so I was relieved when information started to come back to me.

'Kathy, does it say in the book this person is Zoroastrian at all?' I could only think of two possible reasons for this unexpected light show, and Zoroastrianism was one of them.

'It doesn't say anything,' she said. 'But what made you think of that?'

Zoroastrians from Parsee or Persian descent have one of the most interesting and elaborate death rituals in the world – the famed 'Towers of Silence'. Because those of Zoroastrian faith believe that the decaying corpse can contaminate the elements (especially sacred are Earth and Fire), their traditional method of disposal in India is to allow the deceased to be defleshed or 'excarnated', usually by vultures, from these special towers. The process should leave only bones which are bleached by the sun, usually once a year has passed, and pushed into an ossuary pit in the middle of the tower. (Humans during the Neolithic era practised funerary cannibalism for similar reasons. It was seen as more respectful to consume our dead rather than leave them in the dirt or burn them – a case of 'better in than out'.) In the UK at the moment there are no such towers, so Zoroastrians usually opt to be cremated and their ashes interred in a place specific to their religion: part of Brookwood Cemetery in Surrey. Brookwood is the largest cemetery in the UK, created in 1852 specifically for the Necropolis Railway to convey the dead from London to the outskirts. At the time, the city was so full of corpses people were literally tripping over them. The Necropolis train, unbelievably, had first-, second- and third-class tickets for the coffins – and they were, of course, all one way tickets.

Zoroastrian rituals do frequently involve fire, just not in the usual form of cremation, leading some people to call them 'fire worshippers'. According to some information, after a death a fire is lit and kept burning for three days. I surmised that this torch was some form of 'proxy fire' to be kept turned on and to stay with the deceased for the next few days. I explained this to the girls, adding, 'Also, there are two sacred garments associated with Zoroastrians: the *sudreh* and *kusti*.' I opened the bag further and said, 'Look. The *sudreh* is a sacred shirt, like a white vest, symbolising purity and renewal. The *kusti* is a long cord tied round the waist. It has seventy-two strands, symbolising the seventy-two chapters of their holy book.' Both of these objects were present on the deceased, so the mystery, it seemed, had been solved.

As I closed the bag, leaving the torch on, Roxy said, 'That's a bit like the Sikhs with their Kesh, Kangha, Kara, Kirpan and Kachera, isn't it?'

'Yeah, a lot like that,' I agreed. She was referring to the five sacred objects of Sikhism: the bangle, uncut hair, dagger, shorts and wooden comb. 'I'll buy you a pint later if you can tell me which one is which though,' I added, while winking at Kathy, who looked pretty puzzled. It was clear she had no idea what we were talking about but, as a trainee, she had begun her journey and would learn just as much as we had, in time.

I had seen a light associated with death before, but in a different context. In the Jewish tradition, for example, the deceased are not supposed to be left alone right up until the funeral: candles are lit around the body and the deceased should be accompanied by someone at all times as a sign of respect. These guards or keepers are known as *shomerim* and act in a similar way to those who carry out the Perpetual Adoration of the Blessed Sacrament: they don't leave the deceased's side until someone else comes to relieve them. It's a beautiful concept but one that isn't practical in the modern era. Unfortunately, when a Jewish person dies and they're brought to the mortuary they are placed into the fridge like everyone else to ensure the natural process of decay is delayed. Then the porters have to leave, locking up the facility behind them. They can't allow family members to hang around in the closed dark fridge room because it contains multitudes of other deceased patients, as well as private information. A compromise seems to have been created in the form of night lights which I've seen some mortuaries plug into viewing-room wall sockets whenever a Jewish viewing is to take place, then moved to the fridge room once the deceased is placed back in the fridge.

In addition to this, Judaism prohibits any autopsy as the preference is that nothing belonging to the dead should leave the body. But if one is required for legal reasons we have to go ahead and try to facilitate Jewish preferences as much as we can. This is usually fine in the case of organs – as I've explained, they often don't need to be retained. But fluids? This is much more difficult. I have carried out such autopsies with great care, under the watchful eye of rabbis and even family members, trying my absolute best not to spill a drop of blood during the evisceration. If a droplet did land on the deceased or tray I'd use a moist piece of tissue or cotton wool to absorb it and place it immediately into the body cavity. There was no sponging it off and hosing it down the drain. The pathologist also made as little mess as possible, which was such a revelation! They could actually carry out dissections without leaving a bloodbath – who knew?

For those of the Muslim faith, we'd have a compass painted on the floor of the viewing room or a mark on the wall so that we could point the deceased to Mecca, and with some African faiths we allowed huge groups of mourners in at a time. They'd bring rum and pour some on the floor, sometimes all swigging from the bottle and offering it to us. And we had to drink – it was seen as incredibly rude to say no. Those were very good viewings . . .

We had a drawer full of different religious texts for any next of kin from any faith: Judaism, Bahá'í, Hinduism . . . and this is why it's incredibly frustrating when TV shows and films decide to display a 'viewing' in that incredibly clichéd and clinical way I'm sure many are familiar with. Picture the following scene. The family or friend of the decedent has been brought in to view them at him 'morgue'. They are taken into a sterile white or stainless-steel area full of fridge doors and led to one in particular. There, the attendant (whoever they may be representing, sometimes mortuary staff but other times, incorrectly, a pathologist) opens a door and pulls out a tray with a swish. Then they gesture, and say, 'Is this him? I'll give you a minute,' or something along those lines.

This just isn't how we do viewings in the UK. As I mentioned, the fridge room or body store is off limits to the general public and instead we go to a lot of trouble so that family members may see their dead in more comfortable and familiar surroundings.

Once I was fully trained in Liverpool, I began to take part in an evening on-call system – a fairly nightmarish one-week-in-three during which I had to take a pager everywhere with me, even to the gym, to the bath and the toilet. But it was for a good reason: it was for emergencies such as facilitating parents desperate to see recently deceased sons or daughters, and assisting those of a religious persuasion who may require a burial within twenty-four hours. Despite us offering this service, we learned one morning that the previous night a young man had been brought into the mortuary. Because it was so sudden his mother and father, understandably, wanted to view him. However, instead of making use of the on-call service and pager system, the undertakers who brought him in took it upon themselves to do the viewing.

'How hard can it be?' you could almost hear them thinking, 'We've seen how they do it on TV.'

So they took the parents into the fridge room and pulled open a large white door. But because each unit contains several deceased individuals on different shelves the parents were subjected to a view of four pairs of strangers' feet as well as their son's. Then he was pulled out with a theatrical flourish (*swishhhh*), the body bag unzipped (*zzzzzzzzip*), and they saw their son.

Who had just died suddenly of meningitis.

Who was only nineteen years old.

Those parents should never have had to go through that when we trained individuals could have at least made the experience slightly less traumatic with our relatively comfortable room. Such a thoughtless thing to do, and all because of TV stereotypes.

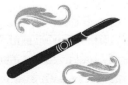

Knowing that I hadn't 'seen a soul' that day didn't stop me thinking of them. I found myself reflecting upon life and death and what it all really meant more and more during my last year as an APT. It wasn't that I was actually considering being a nun or beginning to believe in the afterlife, it was more a case of finding my own happiness; my true path. I'd worked so hard from childhood to enter the death profession and I'd had a great eight-year career so far, so it was scary to entertain the idea of doing something else – but I considered the Buddhists and their conviction that things must change. Just like everyone's journey, mine had had highs and lows. There had been obstacles: I'd encountered people who perhaps caused me to lose some enthusiasm for what I was doing; I'd had no time for any creative pursuits, which I realised was important for me; and I was feeling fragile again, just like I had when I first moved to London. I questioned myself a lot. What am I *doing*? What do I actually *want*? Do I even want to live in London or should I move home? In all the years I'd been working in mortuaries nothing much had improved, nothing had changed. Denise had moved out of our flat and I was back to living with strangers. I was single again, and still didn't feel like I had close friends. Every day, even with the variety in cases or pathologists or undertakers, was inevitably the same.

Albert Einstein is widely credited with saying 'the definition of insanity is doing the same thing over and over again, but expecting different results'. Whether he actually said that is debatable, but the sentiment is true. What would change if *I* didn't make a change? Perhaps I could sell my soul to the Devil for talents and riches beyond my wildest dreams. Perhaps I could somehow earn enough money to go travelling around South America and South East Asia? Problem was, I didn't believe in the Devil and I didn't have the patience to save up thousands of pounds.

So I did something as dramatic as I could think of. Despite always wanting to work in a mortuary, despite my years of voluntary work and the hours I'd put into this career, despite the fact my job seemed to be the thing that defined me, I just knew something had to change.

I quit.

And I went to live in a convent, because I wanted some peace and quiet. I wanted time away from my pain and the man who had caused it, as well as the people I saw daily who reminded me of that. I wanted time away from other people in general; the solitude actually to think about my next move without the distraction of a million other things: the loudspeaker at the tube station; the Halal butcher over the road who was always determined to chat even when I felt like shit and tried to rush past him; the exes who seemed to find it appropriate, while drunk, to text me in the middle of the night; and even my family, who were concerned I was losing my mind. But I wasn't losing my mind – I knew exactly what I was doing. For the first time I was completely free to rest and try to still my thoughts. If I'd been rich, perhaps I would have gone to a health spa. Perhaps I could have 'found myself' while being massaged to within an inch of my life with luxurious oils, spending hours in a flotation tank and breathing deeply during yoga. But I was not rich and I did not want that kind of interaction. I needed to listen to me and me alone. I spent a few weeks researching and I'd discovered you could stay with nuns for as little as £20 a day. By the end of my first month 'unemployed' I was a tenant at a convent.

For anyone who has watched *Father Ted* or *Sister Act*, there is an idea that staying in a religious institution is like a comedy sketch. I can't speak for every institution, but in my experience it was sometimes *exactly* like that. I had a whale of a time!

I had my own small room with a window, a few pieces of furniture, the electric heater I so adored, and a crucifix on the wall. That was pretty much it.

The nuns observed the Divine Office or Liturgy of the Hours, which is a way of marking the day with constant worship. The first, Nocturns, I'd observed at 5.30 a.m. There was also:

Lauds	7.00 a.m.
Mass	7.30 a.m.
Terce	9.15 a.m.
Sext	12.10 p.m.
None	3.15 p.m.
Vespers	4.30 p.m.
Compline	8.15 p.m.

Meals too were on a timetable: breakfast 8.15 a.m., lunch 12.30 p.m. and supper 6.15 p.m. But I was free to do whatever I desired. I could attend services if I wanted or not bother at all. I could eat all meals, or avoid them, or I could make myself tea and coffee and eat biscuits as much as I wanted. I spent a lot of time in the amazing library, even discovering a copy of one of my favourite pieces of writing, Dante's *Inferno*, from 1903. I found a small ante-room off the library with a fire and two rocking chairs and I wrote in there: ideas for a book, blog posts I might eventually publish, a bucket list of things I wanted to do before I died, and more. There was even an equivalent of *Father Ted*'s Mrs Doyle there in the form of a young Polish girl called Elizabeth. Every night around nine p.m., after Compline, she'd bring a cup of Horlicks or Ovaltine to my room when she knew I was winding down for sleep. I'd never thought it fit to consume hot malted drinks anywhere previously but in a convent it just seemed so right. The combination of the peace, the hot milky beverages and the complete and utter silence were soothing to what I can only assume was my soul.

I'd spent so many years reconstructing other people it was unusual, but nice, to be reconstructing myself.

Father Connolly, the resident priest, was usually at the table at mealtimes. He was from Ireland, wore incredibly thick glasses and snorted snuff. His Irish accent was so thick I could barely understand him so I was very surprised to discover he'd been living mostly in Egypt for sixteen years. In fact, he'd been working on an archaeological dig out there which gave us so much to talk about. I'd never expected to find myself in a convent discussing skeletal remains with an Irish priest whose sweater was covered in excess snuff that had floated down from his nose. He talked about how much he'd loved the air hostesses' uniforms on the way over to Egypt and how he admired someone like Silvio Berlusconi rather than, say, David Cameron because 'at least he had a personality'. It was hilarious how one minute he'd be making us all laugh with lewd tales then the next he'd be discussing torture and martyrdom with utter seriousness, all with snuff around his nose. He was a total character.

For me, being there and trying out the whole experience

meant that I wanted to participate in as many services as I could – I mean, it's not as though I was swamped with other things to do. It blew my mind that I'd usually been to *four* religious services by nine thirty – the time when most people were just considering getting out of bed on a Saturday. Mass was mostly a simple affair and the only one I'd actually go into the main church for, rather than sit in my usual place on the balcony. But on a Sunday it was much more of a spectacle with around three or four visiting priests, and a much longer ceremony. Father Connolly seemed like he was plucking his words from thin air, totally unprepared; the Italian Father Gino was young and suave – a bit too good-looking to be a priest; and ancient Father Paddy sat in a chair on the altar, not moving the whole time. He was like a tiny grey-haired turtle, somehow defying normal human life expectancy. It felt like he had no idea where he was.

One morning at breakfast after Mass, while we were discussing the difference between orange jam and actual marmalade, one of the nuns came in from next door to ask how we all were. There were more of us because it was Sunday and the visiting priests had joined us too. When she got to the practically immobile Fr Paddy, she asked, 'Hello Father Patrick, and how are you?' There was a beat of silence and then, in a very quiet but thick Irish accent, he simply replied, 'Still breathing.'

Fr Gino complained of a bad back so the housekeeper Elizabeth handed him a leaflet for a massage parlour as he was finishing his toast. He was sceptical and said, in broken English, 'But what if ... this ... it kill me?' Then he had concerns that, as a priest, he might go into the 'wrong' type of massage parlour, to which Fr Connolly, of course, said, 'If there's no red light in the window you'll be fine, Gino.'

Also staying at the convent was a woman named Regina. Regina means 'queen', but she didn't look like a queen. I mean this in the best way, but she looked and acted the exact opposite of one: humble and kind. She was short and slightly rounded with dark hair and glasses and always wore an outfit that could have been a uniform. I don't know what she actually did – she was visiting from America as she had always wanted to come to this famous convent and church. I learned from her that there were actually related communities all over the world under the one name and people often visited from one to the next. I wondered if she was a novitiate.

'So what is it you plan to do while you stay here?' she asked me one day in the library. She never asked me why I was there – no one did. It was as though they knew it was my own business and didn't want to pry, just to help.

'I don't have a definite plan,' I replied. 'I suppose I just want to spend some time thinking, reading, writing. Just get some peace and quiet.'

'All good things,' she said. 'But of course the best thing you can do while you're here is spend your time in adoration.'

I thought about that long after I'd left the convent. 'Adoration' means something specific in the Catholic faith – worship and prayer in front of the exposed Blessed Sacrament – but it resonated with me on other levels. The best thing I can do while I'm here on this Earth, perhaps? To adore things: myself, my family and friends, nature, every moment that I was alive, the smallest things like the smell of fresh coffee in the morning, the sound of rain on the window when I didn't have to leave my bed, the endorphin rush after going for a run? All of those things we take for granted and can only appreciate properly when we understand how short our time 'here' is.

I keep saying I 'took the time to think' at the convent, and I really did. I realised I hadn't been getting the time to process anything that happened during my hectic life, and perhaps it's the same for many other people. I had always thought it was enough that I would enter a 'Zen zone' while stitching the deceased or clearing out plugholes in the mortuary sinks; I thought the quiet time during my runs was enough to fully clear my mind. But it wasn't. I was just assimilating each day's events. I wasn't far away enough away from my situation actually to contemplate it.

I thought back to my first mortuary manager, Andrew. So serious. He did very few autopsies unless they were particularly interesting cases, and at the time, as a trainee taking my cues from my trainer, I resented him. It was only now, years later, I realised it had been an amazing experience for me to be thrown in at the deep end and carry out autopsies every single day. I had learned more and worked harder in my three years at the Municipal Mortuary than some other APTs do in ten.

And the men at the Metropolitan Hospital who I had so disliked working with; perhaps they just weren't used to having a female in the workplace and didn't act in a manner I felt was appropriate? And perhaps I was too sensitive after making a dramatic life-change and moving to London with barely a second thought. My GP in Liverpool had told me after my London bombings work that I had post-traumatic stress disorder when I'd simply gone to see him with the flu and a cold sore. 'Why would I have PTSD after working a job I'd wanted to do since I was a child,' I'd thought, 'especially on such an important case?' But he may have been right: during those two weeks in the capital I'd been sleep-deprived, constantly under media scrutiny and right in the middle of the biggest terror attack we'd ever seen. Perhaps, then, returning to London and working with Danny and Chris again brought it all screaming back to me without me realising?

I thought back to St Martin's where I'd eventually found myself doing more paperwork than post-mortems and it had irritated me. I couldn't see it at the time but all that managerial experience, and organising funerals and viewings, meant I hit the ground running when applying for other jobs later on. I'd felt hurt by my female colleagues by what I felt was their lack of support after my miscarriage and subsequent fragility. But perhaps it hadn't been personal? Perhaps they never knew the full story about what happened.

All these things I looked at from a different angle once I was finally far enough away. And I let them all go.

My observation of Thomas and Tina's relationship – two mortuary professionals, happily married – inspired me to do something no one else had done before: create a dating site specifically for death professionals. My mum helped me to come up with the title: 'Dead Meet'. I knew some people in the industry might find it macabre and others hilarious, but I was on my *own* path now. Inspiration was hitting me from all angles and I knew that everything up until that point had 'happened for a reason', as they say. Whatever direction I was being pushed in by fate, I intended to follow it. I then began a blog to ensure that my opinions on the death industry and death theory, as well as the display of human remains, were in the public sphere. I kept up to date with academic research, even found my niche area in the strange connection between anatomical displays and the sexual gaze (i.e. the connections between sex and death) and started a Master's degree. I began to flourish; not like the moonflower this time and perhaps not quite yet finding the sun, but more like my favourite line from the book I'd spent so much time reading at the convent. In the Inferno, Dante finally escapes the Underworld and the series ends:

"Now we came out and once more saw the stars"

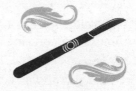

A viewing room containing someone's loved one becomes sacred whether it's called a Chapel of Rest or simply a facility, different from when it's empty and an exhausted or depressed APT like me has slept in it. A church, whether a service is going on or not, is a place you don't swear or mess about in. A human body, whether it's gone through an accidental death or a natural one, deserves the same respect as its neighbour. Anything can be considered sacred if we think of it that way. Regardless of any religious leanings I had, that was not what I was at the convent for. It was there that I learned the meaning and value of 'adoration' and 'contemplation'. It was there that I experienced my own symbolic death and realised how I actually wanted to live. It was there I was able to see the stars.

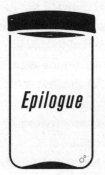

The Angel's Share

There is nothing more comforting than walking into my museum office on a Monday morning. After carrying my bags up a flight of stone steps it's nice to take out my heavy, familiar key, unlock the door and enter my home away from home. After flipping up the blind and turning on the lights, I breathe a small sigh of satisfaction before hanging my coat up and surveying my surroundings. Keeping me company in the office are two severed plastic heads which medical students used to practise their resuscitation skills on. The heads have been decapitated, but despite this they both wear the expressions of satisfied ecstasy common to CPR dummies: half-closed eyes and demi-smiles concealing secrets only they know. In fact, all CPR dummies have the same face as they are modelled on one individual, *L'Inconnue de la Seine* – the unknown woman of the Seine. The woman in question, who was never identified, was assumed to have been a drowning victim. After she was found in the famous Paris river in the 1800s, her body was exhibited in the Paris Morgue. Her death mask, taken in plaster by a smitten pathologist, was popular as wall art in homes from 1900 onwards, a bit like those three flying ducks you'd see adorning walls in the 1970s, and was used to create the face of the Resusci Anne CPR doll in 1958, a tradition which still continues.

Also in my office is the skeleton of a cat – a gift from a colleague – a chocolate spine and a whole shelf of blank-eyed human skulls waiting to be catalogued. Body parts of various styles, shapes and flavours surround me, so I'm not alone and I'm definitely not lonely. I have no office cohabitant enquiring about my weekend activities, which means there's no need to admit my *Murder, She Wrote* marathon to anyone. When I go to grab the fresh coffee for my cafetière I know it will be in the fridge where I left it because there's no one else here to drink it, and if I want to turn on the faux fire in the wooden fireplace I can do so without someone else complaining that they're too warm. Having worked in freezing mortuaries for eight years I have a serious heat fetish and am thrilled to be in control of my own thermostat at last.

The walls in the office may be a bizarre shade of salmon pink and the cupboards may be full of things I daren't move because the twenty years' worth of dust would give me an asthma attack, but this is a little paradise for me. I think Evelyn Waugh put it best in *The Loved One* when he said of his pet-cremating protagonist, Dennis, 'There at the quiet limit of the world he experienced a tranquil joy.' Working with the dead places me on the fringes of normal human experience, but it doesn't have to be traumatic: my quiet limit of the world now involves the scent of coffee, the sound of forties and fifties music, and five thousand parts of deceased individuals who are quite literally resting in pieces.

Bart's Pathology Museum is not a mortuary, yet somehow my eight-year stretch on the front line of contemporary death led me here, to the sanctity of these four noble walls. St Bartholomew's Hospital is the oldest in Europe to exist on the same site – it has been at West Smithfield, London, since 1123. The hospital was originally a monastery founded by a monk, Rahere, gradually expanding into a larger building with extra space for beds, a medical school, research facilities and more.

It was here that William Harvey conducted his pioneering studies on the circulatory system in the seventeenth century. Here, too, Percivall Pott developed important principles of modern medicine in the eighteenth century, such as demonstrating that a certain cancer may be caused by an environmental carcinogen. And here, in the late nineteenth century, Ethel Bedford Fenwick created a nationally recognised certificate for nursing, advancing the profession in the process. As a result of the hospital's rich history, every time building works are carried out reams and reams of skeletons are found buried deep in the ground, some of which are a thousand years old.

Bart's is also the place where Sherlock Holmes meets Dr Watson in the first of the Sherlock books. It's even been said that Conan Doyle wrote *A Study in Scarlet* in my very office. (Although I doubt the walls were salmon pink back then. Perhaps they were scarlet?) And now I am honoured to be a part of such an illustrious institution. As a lover of vintage fashion, old detective novels and anything antique I really don't think I could have ended up anywhere more perfect.

My first day at Bart's was 31 October 2011, rather apt given it was Halloween and most people would consider a place such as this, with its anatomical specimens and skeleton-filled floor, to be quite spooky. Halloween was originally the festival of Samhain (pronounced *sow*-en), a pagan celebration during which we honoured our dead, and this museum is a place in which the dead are honoured. Personally, I don't think the museum is any spookier than a church. In fact, like a church, the cavernous Victorian museum is a sacred space; a sanctuary. Rows upon rows of specimens, like pews of dignified worshippers, are embraced by three storeys' worth of Victorian Portland stone, and are only just protected from the unpredictable British weather by a lantern ceiling of fragile glass. Six huge copper-shaded lights hang down from the crossbeams like censers, and the 'pulpit' at the front – the lectern – has been host to a slew of esteemed speakers who've regaled thousands of visitors with fascinating 'sermons'. It is a cathedral built to protect the relics within and dedicated to sharing knowledge with its congregation – knowledge of the history, diagnosis and healing of disease.

In the *Pharsalia*, an epic poem about the civil war in Rome written by Lucan in AD 61–65, much space is dedicated to the activities of the terrifying necromancer and witch Erictho. She was described as fearsome and disgusting, unkempt and haggard, with skin as pale as bone and hair as black as night. She was said to inhabit deserted tombs and to communicate with corpses; a woman so terrible that even the wolves and vultures fled from her. Yet her talents were unsurpassed when it came to raising the dead, so politicians and military men would seek her out for her divinatory powers, men such as the General Sextus Pompey, who was fighting

Caesar's formidable armies. In one elaborate passage, Erictho reanimates a fresh corpse to command it to divine the future. After a magical ritual of exhuming the corpse, opening its body cavity and filling it with a vile yet magical mixture,

> at once the congealed gore warmed up, soothed the black wounds and ran into the veins and the extremities of the limbs. As the blood struck them the organs beneath the chill breast quivered and life, creeping anew into the innards that had forgotten it, mingled itself with death.

I don't go around digging up corpses in an attempt to enter into discourse with them, despite my obvious enthusiasm for my job, but in some ways my role in the museum is the same. My aim is metaphorically to bring the dead back to life in order to hear their stories once more, or even interpret their prophecies of the future.

Each day at Bart's my process is similar to when I worked in mortuaries. As an APT I used to 'read' the flesh of the deceased by sight and touch, like words and Braille, to compose the story of the end of their lives. I read bruises, scars, tattoos and medical interventions on the parchment of the skin to help the pathologist describe the deceased's last moments and determine cause of death. Here in the museum, like Erictho coaxing silent spirits of the dead back into their withered flesh, I try to build a narrative of each individual, resurrect them from their medical origins and plunge them into that liminal space between history, public health, literature and art. Whether a year old or a hundred years old, everybody has a story.

Before I was appointed as sole staff member, the museum

had begun to fall into disrepair; for years it had only been in use by medical students and doctors. Initially, my main task was to go through all five thousand anatomical specimens and repair, clean or rearrange them depending on what was necessary. Because the Human Tissue Authority doesn't govern human remains over a hundred years old I started by going through every single pot and checking their ID numbers and dates against my catalogues. If they were older than a hundred years I brought them down to the ground floor, meaning we'd eventually be able to allow the general public to see them – something that hadn't happened in the museum's history.

The age of these specimens opened up a whole new world of pathological conditions we barely see any more, which made them so much more special and unique. Chimney Sweep's Cancer of the scrotum, for example, affected the males in that particular vocation, as the name suggests. It is a sad fact that during the 1700s and 1800s young boys were forced to clean chimneys naked, and because the skin of the scrotum can be fairly wrinkly the soot would stick inside the crevices. Eventually, around when the boys hit puberty, a wart-like sore would form on their scrotums, which was often mistaken for something sexually transmitted. The sweeps used to use blades or sharp pieces of wood to try and 'scrape off' the wart. Their attempts were futile and eventually the wart would grow to cover a larger area of skin because it was, in fact, a carcinoma. This link was made by Bart's own surgeon Percivall Pott – the first to connect a malignant disease with an occupation – in effect making him the person responsible for our Health and Safety at Work Acts. We have three examples of these scrotums in the collection and you can see every wrinkle and pubic hair. Even though they're fragments, dissociated from the deceased, the narrative that accompanies the specimens in the pots makes them whole: they're not objects, they're subjects with colourful and lively tales; when you read about them and examine each mark upon the flesh, the human story comes through. To me, it feels like each specimen is a post-mortem from the past, and I'm still reading the histories of the individuals as I used to, although instead of them being sent to me from the local Coroner I'm digging them up from years gone by.

We as a team began to put on events, and the museum's reputation began to grow. It was recognised as a huge resource, an opportunity to create a space for unique engagement of the public with pathology as well as a hub of research. Suddenly, no two days were the same and I began to receive more unusual requests: a famous fashion designer wanted to do a photoshoot in the museum; artists wanted to display their work in the beautiful exhibition space; heavy rock bands wanted to do special acoustic music sets among the specimens. The museum, like myself, had been reborn.

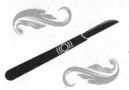

The phone rang one morning as I was taking a sip of coffee and I answered: 'Hello, Pathology Museum.' (It had taken a long time for me to stop saying 'Hello, Mortuary'.)

The voice on the other end of the line was a woman from the press office and she could barely contain her excitement.

'Oh my *God*, do you know who wants to come and visit?' She didn't even give me a chance to answer before she squealed, 'Bradley Cooper!'

I was silent for a minute before saying, 'Hmm, OK.' Famous Hollywood star and heart-throb Bradley Cooper? I mean, I *guess* I could fit him in, but there is a heart to be re-potted, a kidney that's started leaking all over the second level, and I just found another uterus in one of the cupboards that I need to search out in the catalogue. Still, an hour showing off the specimens and a coffee with Bradley might be nice. All in a day's work.

Bibliography

The First Cut
Fisher, Pam, 'Houses for the dead: the provision of mortuar
ies in London, 1843–1889', *The London Journal, 34* (2009),
1–15

1. Information: 'Media Most Foul'
Dick, Philip K., 'How To Build A Universe That Doesn't Fall
Apart Two Days Later' (1978)
Lynch, Thomas, *The Undertaking: Life Studies from the
Dismal Trade*, W. W. Norton and Company (1997)

2. Preparation: 'Grief Encounters'
Churchill, Winston, on his 75th birthday in 1949

3. Examination: 'Judging a Book by its Cover'
Neruda, Pablo, 'Ode To A Naked Beauty/Beautiful Nude'
Gale, Christopher P. and Mulley, Graham P, 'Pacemaker
explosions in crematoria: problems and possible solutions',
Journal of the Royal Society of Medicine (2002), 95(7):
353–355

Phillips, A.W., Patel, A.D. and Donell, S. T., 'Explosion of Fixion(R) humeral nail during cremation: Novel "complication" with a novel implant', *Injury Extra* Volume 37, Issue 10 (2006), 357–358

Roach, Mary, *Stiff*, W. W. Norton and Company (2003)

Richardson, Ruth, *Death, Dissection and the Destitute*, Routledge (1988)

Davies, Rodney, *Buried Alive*, Robert Hale (2000)

4. Difficult Examination: 'Pulp Fiction'

Goll, Iwan, (1891–1950) 'Teenage Angst': Placebo, Sony/ATV Music Publishing LLC, 1996. By Brian Molko, Stefan Olsdal and Robert Schultzberg

Quigley, Christine, *The Corpse: A History*, McFarland and Co., (1996)

5. Penetration: 'Rose Cottage'

Attar, Farid ud-Din, (c. 1145–c. 1221), *The Conference of the Birds*

Shillace, Brandy, *Death's Summer Coat: What the History of Death and Dying Can Tell Us About Life and Living*, Elliott and Thompson, (2015)

Nuland, Sherwin B., *How We Die*, Random House (1993) 'When masturbation can be fatal: The practice of auto-erotic asphyxia is often concealed by a coroner's verdict', Monique Roffey, *The Independent* (1993) http://ind.pn/29wIbqB

Bronfen, Elizabeth, *Over Her Dead Body*, Manchester University Press (1992)

6. Thoracic Block: 'Home Isn't Where the Heart Is
Autumn, Emilie, *The Asylum for Wayward Victorian Girls*,
   The Asylum Emporium (2009)
Coronary Heart Disease Statistics: http://bit.ly/1VkqriW

7. Abdominal Block: 'Pickled Punks'
'In Bloom', Nirvana, Warner/Chappell Music, Inc., BMG
   Rights Management US, LLC, 1991. By Kurt Cobain
Ebenstein, Joanna, *The Anatomical Venus*, Distributed Art
   Publishers (2016)

8. The Head: 'Losing my Head'
'Break the Night with Colour': Richard Ashcroft, Kobalt
   Music Publishing, 2006. By Richard Ashcroft
Collins, Kim A, 'Postmortem Vitreous Analyses', Medscape
   (2016)
   http://bit.ly/2mb8jfT
Maning, Frederick Edward, *Old New Zealand* (1983)

9. Fragmented Remains 'Bitsa'
'Bitsa', BBC, 1992. By Peter Charlton
'Genitals Stolen in Morgue', Mervyn Naidoo, *BBC, 7 June 2015*
   http://bit.ly/2mblLjQ
'Decomposition Rats Between Humans, Pigs May Vary
   Wildly', Seth Augenstein, *Forensic Magazine,* 5 March
   2016
   http://bit.ly/2lJnD2q
'Body parts left over from operations should be used to
   help train police dogs', Martin Evans, *The* Telegraph, 3
   February 2016
   http://bit.ly/1NPLShV

10. Reconstruction: 'All the King's Men'

Hawking, Stephen, *A Brief History of Time*, Bantam Press (1988)

Bones without Barriers: http://boneswithoutbarriers.org/

'What You Need to Know About Skin Grafts and Donor Site Wounds', Pauline Beldon, *Wounds International* http://bit.ly/2lJd5jS

Chin, Gail, 'The Gender of Buddhist Truth: The Female Corpse in a Group of Japanese Paintings', *Japanese Journal of Religious Studies*, Vol 25, No 3/4 (1998), 277–317 http://bit.ly/2moYFCi

11. Chapel of Rest: 'Sister Act'

McCarthy, Jenny, *Love, Lust & Faking It: The Naked Truth About Sex, Lies, and True Romance*, HarperCollins Publishers (2010)

Acknowledgements

Firstly I have to give a huge thanks to my fantastic agent Robyn Drury for recognising the potential in such a rough diamond and making it shine – that applies to *me* as well as the book – and to the whole team at Diane Banks Associates who have been incredibly supportive.

Thanks also to the team at Little, Brown for believing in my story and helping it become a reality: they are the midwives to this 'book birth' and I couldn't have done it without them guiding me every step of the way, telling me when I needed to 'breathe' and metaphorically wiping my brow. Special thanks go to my editor Rhiannon Smith who spurred me on with every possible encouraging gif of *Midsomer Murders* she could find because, yes, that's the kind of encouragement I respond to. And thanks to Jack Smyth for the beautiful cover, which I'm very happy for this book to be judged by!

Special thanks and all my love goes to my supportive and incredibly patient fiancé, Jonny Blyth, who is my rock. He was probably so tired of my repetitive refrain: 'I can't watch a film – I HAVE A BOOK TO WRITE!' and 'I can't go to the barbecue – I HAVE A BOOK TO WRITE!' but now the book is here and I'm sure he feels like a proud baby-daddy. He should, I couldn't have done this without him.

My family are used to me being a crazy nutter who takes on far too much at once, but this time I worried them half to death by writing a book at the same time as everything else I was working on. Thanks to my mum, Collette, and my brother, Ryan, for always being at the other end of the phone or at the station to pick me up when it all got a bit too much and I headed up North for lots of comforting carbs with gravy. And a proper brew.

So much gratitude goes to the wonderful Les and Margaret Blyth for their love and kindness. Thank you for taking in another stray and being so supportive.

And I don't know what I would have done without my mentor, role model and Fairy Godmother Cathy Long who was always there to listen to me over a bottle of prosecco in our favourite London restaurant.

Massive thanks to my friends who were helping me through the process even when they didn't know they were: Heather Lower, Emma Thomas, Joanna Hornby, Kerry Hughes, Georgina Bond, Debbie Nathan, Hannah Gosh, Helen Flood and Jane Langley. I really hope I haven't missed anyone out because they WILL kill me, and many of them also know how to get away with it!

Professional gratitude goes to Christian Burt and the rest of the AAPT for procedural updates. Also thanks to Dr Anna Williams who was my anthropology teacher and now champions Body Farms in the UK as she was always happy to talk body parts. And Toni Woodward who was my enucleation teacher and was always happy to talk eyeballs.

A book – like a body – is made up of many parts and I want to thank everyone who follows me, supports me and encouraged me through tough times on social media. Thanks to you all the parts came together and this book is alive, ALIVE!